M. The great Gallery.
N. Vaulted Corridores.
O. Little Courts.
P. Little dining Room
Q. Lesser Closets.
R. Dressing Rooms.
S. Little Appartments
T. Grand Court.
V. Gardens.
W. Little Ante. or waiting

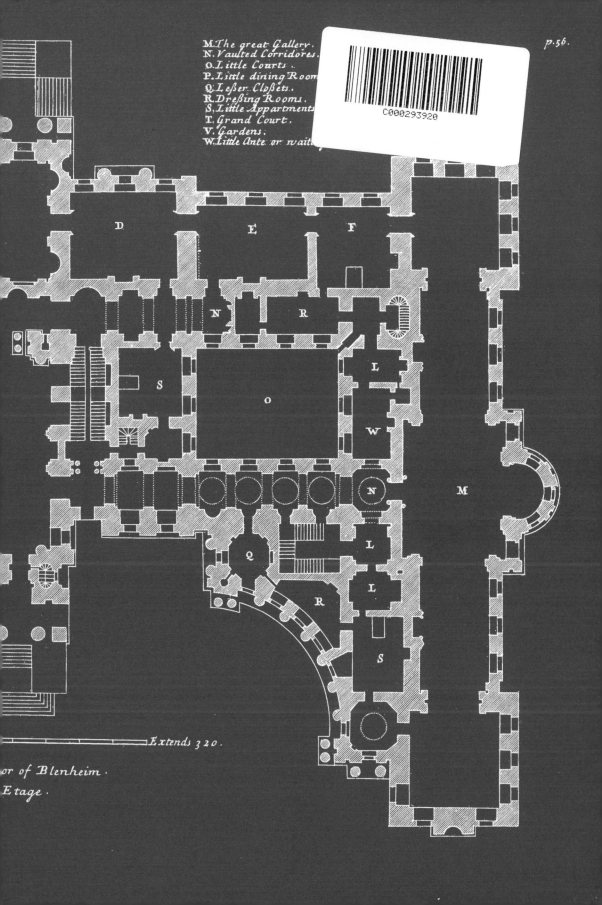

D   E   F

N   R

S

O

L

W

N

M

Q

R   L

L

S

Extends 320.

or of Blenheim.
Etage.

A
PASSION
FOR
FASHION

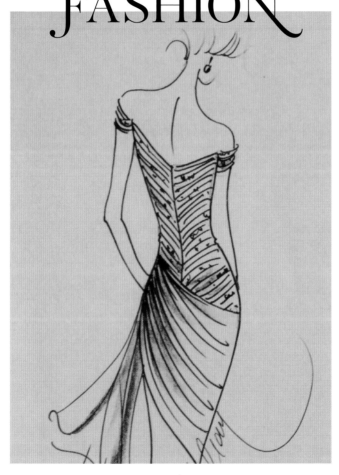

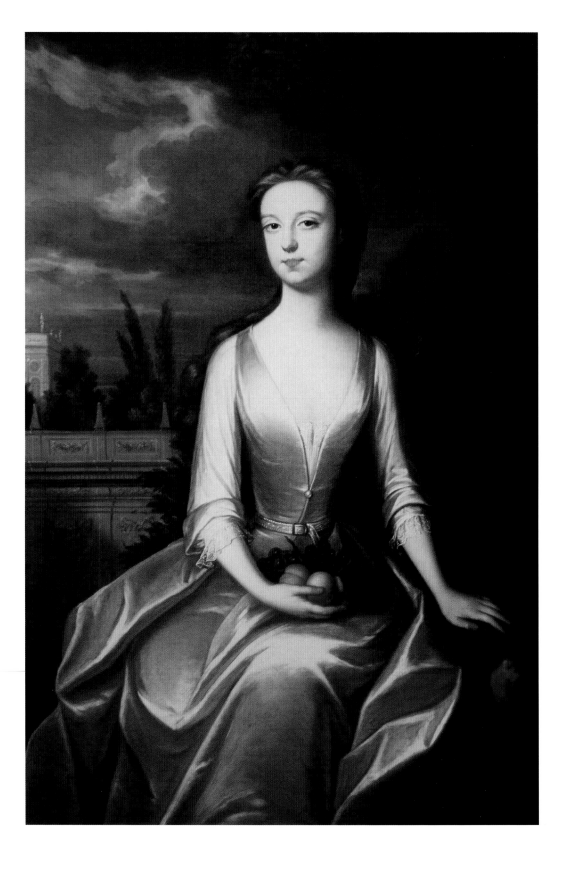

A PASSION FOR FASHION

300 YEARS OF STYLE AT BLENHEIM PALACE

Antonia Keaney

UNICORN

To the Family of Five (Plus!)

and

my Big Brother...
Peter Cosentino
1951–2018

Published in 2019 by
Unicorn, an imprint of Unicorn Publishing Group LLP
5 Newburgh Street
London
W1F 7RG

www.unicornpublishing.org

Text © Antonia Keaney
Images © see picture credits

ISBN 978-1-912690-48-0

10 9 8 7 6 5 4 3 2 1

Designed by Jonathan Christie
Printed in Turkey for Jellyfish

Contents

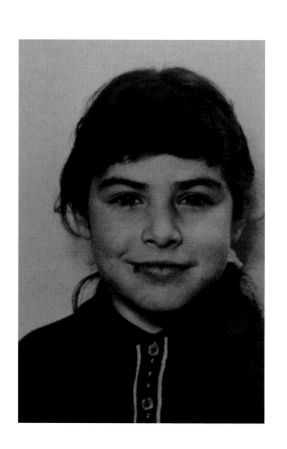

Putting on a show
at Blenheim Palace

It is not entirely predictable from this photograph of me as a seven-year-old that one day I would be tasked with creating an exhibition at Blenheim Palace that looked at the fashions and foibles of some of the great – and not quite so great – people who have been connected with Blenheim in one way or another over the past 300 years.

I remember the day of the photograph so vividly: it was the annual school photo and I had had the misfortune to develop a cold sore. My mum always tied my unruly hair into two tight plaits and, with the help of copious amounts of spittle, managed to bind the ends with wide, blue ribbon.

Having what I now recognise as a slightly obstinate streak, I decided that on this occasion I would wear my hair down: a treat reserved for birthdays. As my turn approached to take a seat in front of the photographer, I panicked and desperately attempted to re-plait my hair. Needless to say, it was not a huge success and the end result was a messy ponytail. Imagine my parents' delight (not) when I came home bearing this particular photograph.

And so it was with *A Passion for Fashion*: plans were made, discarded, revamped. Panic set in, sleepless nights were endured, barefaced cheek was used to achieve my goals, and once or twice things were mislaid or abandoned, including, strangely enough, a brand new suitcase.

Was the end product worth all the angst? Absolutely! As with the photo, something unique and memorable emerged: something from which much was learnt, treasured, savoured and always remembered with a smile.

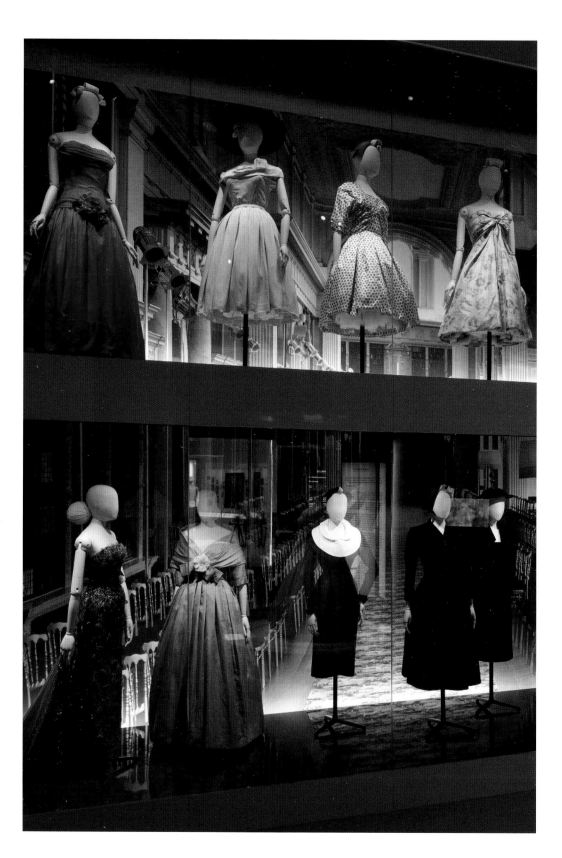

Introduction

Based on a recent Blenheim exhibition of the same name, *A Passion for Fashion* is a very personal, behind-the-scenes look at what is involved in putting on a show in the Palace and at some of the clothes, underclothes, shoes and accessories worn by many of the more colourful characters in Blenheim's 300-year history – not least the twice prime minister of Great Britain, Winston Churchill, whose premature birth in a modest room is one of the many things for which the Palace is famous.

The role that arsenic, lead, mercury and mousetraps played in creating the must-have look of the day is examined, as are adult and children's fashions from the eighteenth and nineteenth centuries. Contemporary styles from renowned designers including Christina Stambolian, Stephen Jones, Christian Louboutin and, most recently of all, Dolce & Gabbana also feature, as do the fabulous 1950's fashion shows by the House of Dior.

A Passion for Fashion brings 300 years of Blenheim style to life.

Left:
Dior in Britain - courtesy of the Victoria and Albert Museum. The backdrop to these exquisite Dior dresses is an image of the Long Library at Blenheim Palace when it was being used to launch the Dior S/S 17 Cruise collection in May 2016

CHAPTER 1

Pink for a Boy!

'…while blue, which is more delicate and dainty is prettier for the girl'

Earnshaw's Infants' Department, June 1918

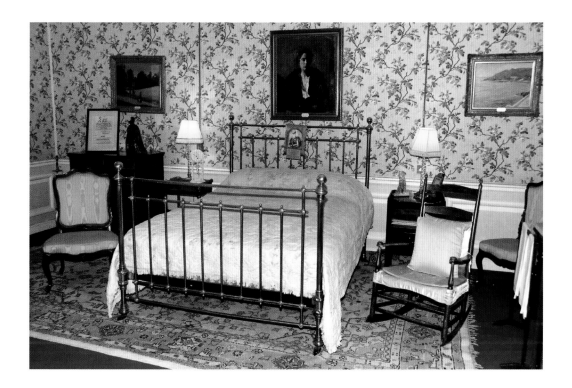

Blenheim Palace is famous for many things, but one of its leading claims to fame is that it happens to be the birthplace of a certain Winston Leonard Spencer-Churchill: twice prime minister of Great Britain and accomplished writer, artist and sometime bricklayer.

His parents, Lord Randolph Spencer-Churchill and American socialite, Jennie Jerome, met at Cowes Week in August 1873. Theirs was a whirlwind romance and Randolph was so besotted that he proposed to Jennie after their second meeting. Randolph's parents, the 7th Duke and Duchess of Marlborough, were not quite as enamoured by the whole idea and initially refused to give their blessing. This was but a minor hitch as far as Randolph was concerned, and eventually the desired blessing was obtained and the happy couple were married in April 1874, less than a year after they had first met.

Randolph and Jennie's style credentials were impeccable. Jennie was always at the leading edge of fashion and a fearless horsewoman at a time when women wore tightly corseted, two-piece outfits in which to ride side-saddle. Randolph, a budding politician and part of the Prince of Wales's set (right up until he tried to blackmail the royal to prevent a Spencer-Churchill family scandal), was always immaculately turned out and sported a luxuriant moustache: to turn up at one's club with a clean-shaved upper lip would be tantamount to appearing without one's trousers!

Randolph and Jennie were frequent visitors

'Randolph sported a luxuriant set of moustaches – to turn up at one's club with a clean shaved upper lip would be tantamount to appearing without one's trousers!'

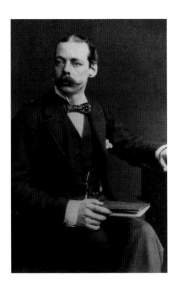

to Blenheim Palace – it was after all Randolph's family home – and it was on one of these visits that the impatient future prime minister put in a premature appearance.

The young couple were due at the Palace for a St Andrew's Day Ball. This of course meant that, transport being what it was, their stay would be for several nights. The festivities took place in the magnificent Long Library and, while everyone was enjoying themselves, Jennie unexpectedly went into labour. The household was unprepared for this event and Jennie was made comfortable in a small side room close to the Long Library that had originally belonged to the rather bulldog-faced Dean Barzillai Jones, Chaplain to the 1st Duke of Marlborough and card player extraordinaire.

Jennie's labour progressed and after a number of hours reached its natural conclusion. Randolph proudly recorded that his premature son was 'wonderfully pretty': the first and possibly the last time that Winston

was described using those words.

The future prime minister was born into the Victorian age on 30 November 1874 and began life dressed in baby linen borrowed from the wife of the Woodstock solicitor according to Randolph, or from his Aunt Lilian according to her sister Norah, who was also present at that time. Whichever it was, it was very lucky that there were some on hand.

Visitors to Blenheim can see the room in which Winston was born, and when I was thinking about what to put where for the 2017 *A Passion for Fashion* exhibition, I decided that a way of linking a display with a particular room would be, as far as possible, to reference a particular item or object in the room. This was straightforward in this instance as hanging on the wall in Churchill's birth room is a striking portrait of a rosy-cheeked, Victorian child. With its auburn ringlets, velvet dress and lacy collar, the child could easily be mistaken for a girl. The portrait is most definitely not that of a girl, but rather that of a four-year-old Winston

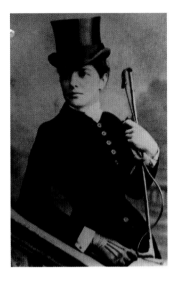 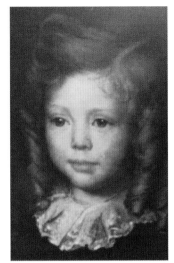 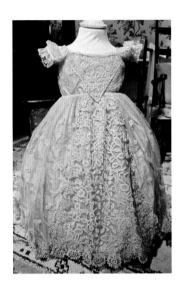

Previous page
Originally Dean Barzillai Jones's room, this was where Winston Leonard Spencer-Churchill was born on 30 November 1874. He was six weeks early and his mother, who was attending a St Andrew's Day Ball at the Palace, is said to have given birth in the room that was being used as a cloakroom! Not an auspicious start one might say.

Opposite page
Randolph Churchill, the younger of the two surviving sons of the 7th Duke and Duchess of Marlborough. He proposed to Jennie Jerome after their second meeting.

Above left
American socialite Jennie Jerome, corseted and ready to ride.

Above centre
Detail from Ayron P. Ward's 1878 portrait of Winston Churchill aged four. The future prime minister wears a velvet dress with lace collar and has beautiful auburn ringlets.

Above right
This beautiful pink dress could have been worn by either a boy or a girl. Gender distinction did not really start to make an appearance until the early twentieth century and at that time pink was the preferred colour for a boy and blue for a girl.

Leonard Spencer-Churchill.

Winston was a Victorian child and the tradition in his family – as it was in many Victorian families – was not to breech the boys or to cut their hair for the first time until they were five years old. He was no exception to this and, once he had passed his fifth birthday, his flowing gowns and dresses were replaced by breeches and jackets, and his beautiful auburn curls were cut but, luckily for us, preserved by his doting parents (or his beloved Nanny Everest) and now hang framed in the room of his birth.

In 1874 there was no distinction between favoured colours for boys and girls and so it was not out of the ordinary for boys to be dressed in pink. Gender distinction did not really start to make an appearance until the early twentieth century and at that time pink was the preferred colour for a boy and blue for a girl.

One of the earliest references to this gender distinction appeared just before the end of the First World War, in June 1918, in an edition of the trade magazine, *Earnshaw's Infants' Department*: 'The generally accepted rule is pink for the boys and blue for the girls…pink being a more decided and stronger colour is more suitable for the boy, while blue, which is more delicate and dainty is prettier for the girl.'

The objective, I fear, was to encourage gullible new parents to rush out to buy the appropriate colour-coordinated wardrobe for their infant, rather than just handing down clothes and using whatever fitted.

This preference persisted until the 1940s, when it was reversed and boys began to be dressed in blue and girls in pink. Fortunately today the gender association has been diluted somewhat – although perhaps girls have the wider choice – yet at one level the pink/blue preference is still so entrenched that, while baby girls are dressed in most colours, it is now relatively unusual to see a baby boy dressed in pink.

If you were to look in the many trunks stored away on the private side of the Palace, which is still inhabited by the present Duke of Marlborough, you would come across numerous dresses, smocks and nightgowns, all of them in white, and fashioned from cotton or linen. This was the staple of any Victorian infant's wardrobe.

Day to day, baby Winston would have been dressed in clothes made from these more utilitarian and practical fabrics: garments that could be boiled and bleached to get them clean, in styles that made nappy changing simpler and that could easily accommodate growing limbs without having to constantly have new clothes made.

Fast forward several years – Winston was sent off to school (with varying degrees of success) and was obliged to wear various uniforms – and it could be argued that this set rather a trend given his years in the army and in government. He was yet to establish his own style.

During the school holidays, Winston was a frequent visitor to Blenheim Palace where he was left under the supervision of his beloved nanny, Mrs Everest, and perhaps his slightly less beloved and far stricter grandmother, the 7th Duchess, while his mother and father were absent, busying themselves with the political arena in which Randolph appeared to have a glittering future.

That said, Winston's grandmother loved and cared for him and arranged for him to learn to ride in the Park at Blenheim. He would have been dressed appropriately – right down to his little leather riding boots – while his pony, Rob Roy, was furnished with a rather splendid

Right
While learning to ride at Blenheim, Winston would have been dressed appropriately, right down to his little leather riding boots.

Far right
Winston's pony, Rob Roy, was furnished with a rather splendid saddle that resembled a leather armchair and virtually guaranteed against the possibility of his taking a tumble during his early rides in the Park.

saddle resembling a leather armchair that virtually guaranteed against the possibility of his taking a tumble during those early rides.

By August 1908 Winston had finished school, passed out at Sandhurst, escaped from the clutches of the Boers during the 1899–1901 war, then managed to make a living for himself by writing before eventually taking his seat as a Member of Parliament for Oldham. His thoughts now turned to romance and he decided that he wished to propose to Clementine Hozier. This was not his first attempt at a marriage proposal: his two earlier attempts had met with as much success as some of his parents' choices of school for him.

This time, it proved to be third time lucky. Winston persuaded Clementine to visit Blenheim Palace for a few days in August 1908. Who could resist a proposal of marriage in such splendid surroundings? Certainly not Miss

Hozier. Although it has to be said that, if it were not for Winston's quick-thinking cousin, the 9th Duke of Marlborough, then Winston may have slept on undisturbed, while Clemmie's patience wore thin as she awaited him in the Great Hall, dressed for their pre-breakfast stroll to the Rose Garden.

On 12 September 1908 Winston and Clemmie were married at St Margaret's, Westminster. They certainly did not believe in long engagements. It was a splendid day and the bride looked radiant, but sadly Winston's wedding apparel fell rather short of the mark. *The Tailor & Cutter* – a trade publication – made no bones about it and referred to Winston's looking like a 'glorified coachman'. Despite his aristocratic background, Winston's choice of clothing was described as one of the 'greatest failures as a wedding garment...ever seen'.

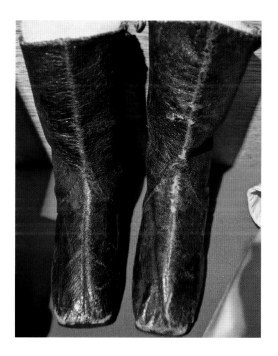

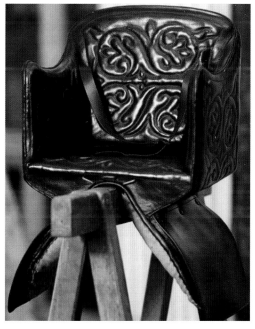

History does not record whether or not the groom donned a going-away outfit, but it can only be hoped that, by the time the newlyweds' train arrived at the now defunct Woodstock railway station, Winston had had the good taste to change into something more appropriate to begin his honeymoon at Blenheim Palace.

Winston moved in exalted circles and numbered the Duke of Westminster among his close friends. He and Clemmie enjoyed the bachelor duke's hospitality at his numerous homes and it was through him that, in 1920, Winston met Coco Chanel. Winston and Coco had various other acquaintances in common, not least Étienne Balsan, the Frenchman with whom Coco Chanel had once had a long relationship. He happened to be the brother of Consuelo Vanderbilt's second husband, Jacques. Consuelo, one-time American heiress and former Duchess of Marlborough, was once

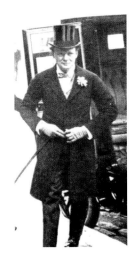

Right
On the occasion of his wedding on 12 September 1908, *The Tailor & Cutter* – a trade publication – described Winston as looking like a 'glorified coachman'. Despite his aristocratic background, Winston's choice of outfit was one of the 'greatest failures as a wedding garment...ever seen'. It begged its readers not to adopt this style!

Below
The Duke of Westminster introduced Winston to Coco Chanel in 1920 and they became firm friends. Despite being a trailblazer in the world of fashion, and the inventor of the Little

Black Dress, Coco Chanel could do very little to influence Winston's sense of style, as demonstrated here in 1929.
© Hugo Vickers

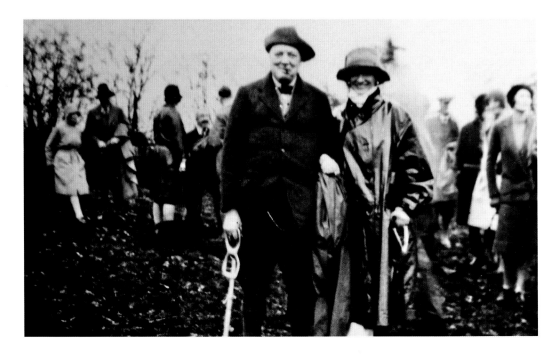

married to Winston's cousin, the 9th Duke of Marlborough.

Coco Chanel and Winston became close friends. She was the Duke of Westminster's acknowledged mistress, as anyone walking through the City of Westminster can still see today by glancing at the monogrammed lamp posts. Sadly, despite being a trailblazer in the world of fashion, and the inventor of the Little Black Dress, Coco Chanel did little to influence Winston's sense of style.

Arguably, the only item that Winston contributed to the world of fashion was the one-piece siren suit. This was a garment based on the overalls that he donned to build walls at his home, Chartwell, and it was happily worn by him in old age, fashioned from many different fabrics, such as velvet, herringbone and tweed: the precursor of the ubiquitous and ever-popular 'onesie'.

Below
Coco Chanel was the Duke of Westminster's acknowledged mistress, as anyone walking through the City of Westminster can still see today by glancing at the monogrammed lamp posts.

Right
Arguably the only item that Winston contributed to the world of fashion was the one-piece siren suit. Based on the overalls he wore to build walls, he owned many variations of it in several different fabrics. The precursor of the ubiquitous and ever-popular 'onesie', perhaps.

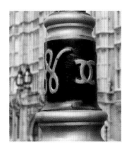

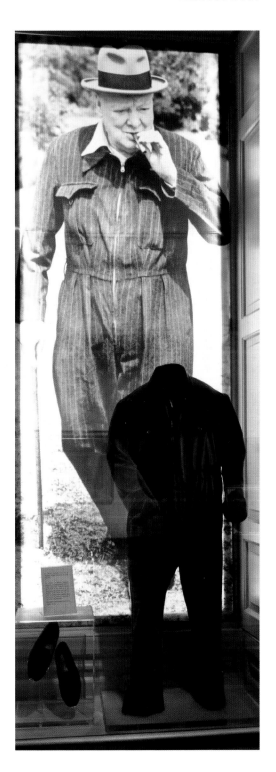

CHAPTER 2

'Enough lice to people a parish'

"An unfortunate state of affairs at a time when the hair creations of the day were kept in place for days or weeks and were notoriously difficult to keep vermin free"

I have always been fascinated by the fact that many names are repeated throughout history, both on a personal level and on a much wider and grander scale. My parents came to England from Italy in the 1950s and I was brought up speaking an archaic southern Italian dialect. Sometimes as I mentally translated things into English, I could not help but be amused at what seemed to be a chronic lack of imagination shown by my ancestors when naming their offspring.

There are so many Pietro Cosentinos (one of whom was my brother) or Rita D'Imperios or Eleanora Lamboglias that a 'sopranome', or nickname, was often applied to distinguish which particular one was being referred to. Eleanora a' copollaianca translates as 'Eleanora White-Hat', Pietro u' fede is 'Peter the Fairy', but poor old Rita clearly got the short straw when she was referred to as Rita a' caccheddá : 'Rita the Shitty' Strangely enough, this is akin to how some of the family names we recognise today originated: Carter, Wheeler, Archer, Fletcher, etc.

I digress, but only slightly. The Spencer family has seen no fewer than four Lady Diana Spencers. I wonder with the Lady Dianas, as with the many Ritas and Pietros, whether any of them share common characteristics. Certainly none of the Dianas appeared to have led charmed lives and, with one exception, they were all very short-lived.

The Spencer-Churchill family – that is, the Dukes of Marlborough – are cousins of the Spencer family of Althorp House in Northamptonshire. The Duke of Marlborough and Earl Spencer share distant great-grandparents in John and Sarah Churchill, the 1st Duke and Duchess of Marlborough.

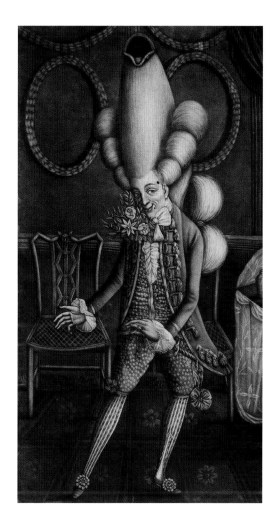

Above
The Macaroni, a real character at the late masquerade, by Philip Dawe, 1773. A very slight exaggeration of eighteenth-century styling for men.

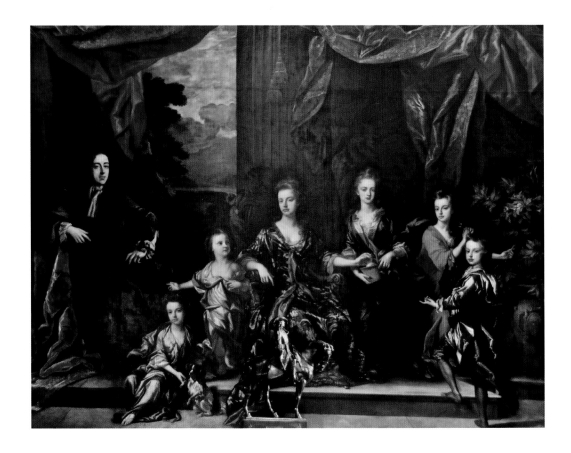

In 1700 one of the 1st Duke's daughters, the fifteen-year-old Anne, married into the Spencer family at Althorp and that is how the connection came about. In fact, the 3rd and 4th Dukes were Spencers and it was the 5th Duke who reintroduced the name 'Churchill' in 1817, to create the family name Spencer-Churchill that is still used today.

The first Lady Diana Spencer (1710–1735) was Anne's daughter and thus granddaughter of Sarah, the 1st Duchess of Marlborough. Diana was one of the few people with whom Sarah did not quarrel: not only because of her sweet nature, but also because of her early demise. Once Lady Diana was married,

Lady Diana was a talented artist and Josiah Wedgewood, recognising a rare talent, went so far as to commission her to create decorative designs for his pottery

to John Russell, later the Duke of Bedford, she and her grandmother exchanged many letters and through these it is possible to learn much about the fashions and fads of the day. It is worth noting that John Russell was not Sarah's first choice of husband for Lady Diana, her favourite granddaughter. She had set her sights much higher, on the Prince of Wales no less. The Prime Minister, Robert Walpole, was none too keen on having a relative of Sarah's on the throne and managed to thwart the duchess's plans.

The China Ante Room at Blenheim houses a marvellous collection of Sevres and Meissen china. It is actually part of a corridor that runs the length of the Palace from east to west, which was created to prevent the Malvern College boys, who were evacuated to Blenheim during the Second World War, from running amok into the duke's private apartments. It is here that evidence of the second – and longest surviving – Lady Diana Spencer (1734–1808) can be found. She was the great-granddaughter of Sarah, the 1st Duchess of Marlborough, and the sister of George Spencer, the 4th Duke of Marlborough.

Lady Diana was a talented artist. Like many genteel ladies of her day, she was taught to draw and paint, but the two self-portraits that hang in the China Ante Room would indicate that Diana had more than a passing talent. In fact, when she was widowed after the death of her second husband, it was Diana's skill at painting and design, coupled with her notoriety, that kept her fed and clothed, as it became increasingly desirable to own a piece of her work. Josiah Wedgwood, recognising a rare talent, even went so far as to commission her to create decorative designs for his pottery.

Lady Diana's first marriage, to Viscount

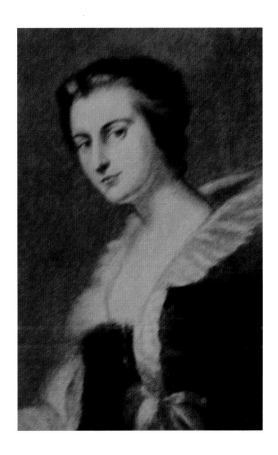

Left
The Marlborough Family, by John Closterman, c. 1694. The Duke of Marlborough and Earl Spencer share distant great-grandparents in John and Sarah Churchill, the 1st Duke and Duchess of Marlborough. In 1700 one of the 1st Duke's daughters, Anne, married into the Spencer family at Althorp and that is how the connection came about.

Above
A self-portrait of Lady Diana Spencer from the 1700s. A talented artist, when she was widowed after the death of her second husband, Topham Beauclerk, it was the income generated by her skill at painting and design that kept her fed and clothed.

'Bully' Bolingbroke, was an abusive one. He owned property and land in Wiltshire and she married him on a whim. Diana did her duty by her husband and presented him with two sons, thus ensuring that the line of succession was safe. Bolingbroke was delighted. He was less than delighted, however, when he realised that his wife was again with child, and that it was none of his doing. The marriage ended in a scandalous divorce because of her 'criminal conversations' (a euphemism for adultery) with the Honourable Topham Beauclerk, the great-grandson of Nell Gwyn, the favoured mistress of Charles II.

In March 1768 the newly divorced Lady Diana married Beauclerk, friend of such eighteenth-century notables as Joshua Reynolds and Samuel Johnson. In his prime he was regarded both as a brilliant conversationalist and as a flamboyant, trendsetting 'dandy' sporting the extreme fashions of the day.

The dandy was a natural progression from the 'macaroni': stylish and fastidiously dressed young aristocrats who, having returned from the 'Grand Tour', spent much of their time in pursuit of their next pair of knee buckles, snuff box, fob watch or other essential accessory. His corseted figure with artificially broad shoulders, layers of lace ruffles at throat and wrist, and striped breeches was easily identifiable, as he appeared in the most fashionable parts of town bedecked with more accessories than you could shake a tasselled stick at.

When thinking about how to illustrate exactly how extreme eighteenth-century men's fashions could be, I hit upon the idea of using a paper sculpture. Mounted on a plain, white

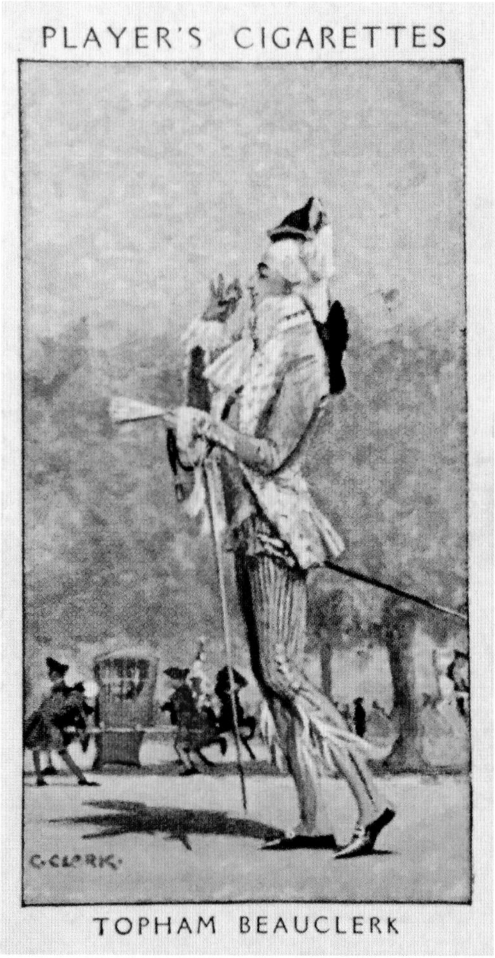

PLAYER'S CIGARETTES

TOPHAM BEAUCLERK

Above
Topham Beauclerk was a brilliant conversationalist and a flamboyant, trendsetting dandy who happily sported the extreme fashions of the day. He is shown here on a John Player's cigarette card from around 1932.

Right
A selection of babies' and children's shoes curated by Althea Mackenzie of the Herefordshire Museum, 2016. The day I visited her to choose from her incredible collection I felt like a very spoilt child let loose in a toyshop.

mannequin, the clothes could be made larger than life and the exaggeration in dress would only be limited by the sculptor's imagination.

Let me backtrack a moment. While researching and planning *A Passion for Fashion*, it quickly became apparent that there would be only a minuscule budget available. There was, therefore, a real danger that our unsuspecting visitors would have very little to see when they actually arrived.

I was fortunate to be chatting with my colleague Gareth Gwilt about this problem when he mentioned an ex-colleague of his, who was very knowledgeable ('what she doesn't know about fashion isn't worth knowing', I think were his exact words) and, a quality not always found in a museum curator or archivist, someone who wanted the collection in her care to be seen, rather than stored away beautifully, never to see the light of day.

This was my first meeting with Althea Mackenzie, and she agreed to help with loans of costumes and accessories from the 1700s right up until the late 1800s, and after various formalities, it only remained for me to point out which items I would like to include in the Blenheim exhibition. The day I visited Althea to choose from her incredible collection I felt like a spoilt child let loose in a toyshop. This is roughly how the conversation proceeded:

Please could I have that...?

Yes...that should be possible...or we have this...

Please could I have both...?

Yes, that should be fine...

And so it was that on a bright winter's day in February 2017, with the help of Head Gardener Hilary Wood and two of her spotlessly clean vans (and two of her spotlessly clean gardeners), we collected over one hundred exquisite items from Althea's keep, all of them wrapped, boxed and labelled with loving care.

But what of the paper sculpture? During my first meeting with Althea she mentioned with great enthusiasm that there was a display of paper costumes in another part of the building. I have to say that my initial reaction was that the costumes sounded a bit odd, but what did I know! The paper clothing, wigs and accessories were created by the amazingly talented Denise Watson and the detail and accuracy with which she had brought the paper costume display to life was stunning. That is how she came to bring

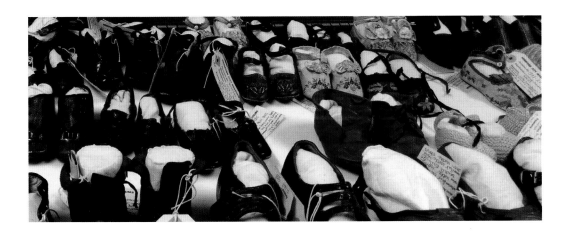

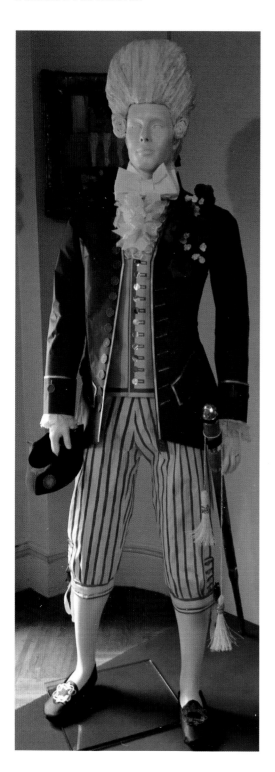

Left

Topham's coat boasted a small collar, fitted sleeves and large decorative buttons. Emerging from each sleeve was a frou-frou of lace ruffles. The carrying of swords was banned in the 1760s, but no self-respecting young man about town would have been seen without his decorated gold-topped walking cane, with or without the tassels.

Right

Denise Watson's design for Topham Beauclerk, 2017.

Far right

The scalp scratcher was a necessity for eighteenth-century men and women of fashion. The fantastic wig creations of the time could stay in place for several days or weeks and were notoriously difficult to keep clean and vermin free.

Topham Beauclerk back to Blenheim after a gap of more than two hundred years.

During his late twenties and early thirties Topham Beauclerk (1739–1780) was at the cutting edge of fashion. Our sculpture was dressed as he would have been, in a close-fitting coat, pleated and flared at the rear with beautifully detailed embroidery. The shape of the coat skirt was less full than it had been in the earlier part of the century, having been gradually cut away to become the 'frock coat' popular in the later 1700s.

Topham's coat boasted a small collar, fitted sleeves and large, decorative buttons. Emerging from each sleeve was a frou-frou of lace ruffles: an echo of those that appeared above his waistcoat, which in turn was topped with an extravagant stock or cravat. Beneath his coat Topham wore a short fitted waistcoat. This was usually the most colourful item in the dandy's

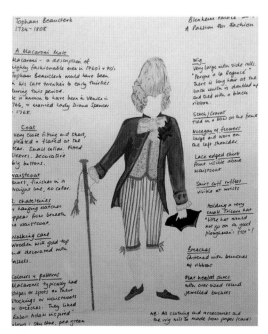

wardrobe (even more than the vivid corsage worn beside his lapel to ward off bad smells) and was made from a sumptuous silk or silk velvet and patterned with stripes or spots: a decoration he would not have been at all reticent about repeating on his breeches and stockings.

Let us not lose sight of the fact that Topham also accessorised his outfits. The carrying of swords was banned in the 1760s, but no self-respecting young man about town would have been seen without his decorated gold-topped walking cane, with or without tassels. With cane in one hand and a small tricorn hat in the other – so small in fact that it would not fit upon his bewigged head – Topham would have cut a fine figure. With all these colours and patterns it is perhaps no wonder that his shoes were relatively plain – hand made, low heeled, black in colour – but even they were decorated or fastened with exquisite silver buckles,

which could be changed at will to update and transform them.

Lady Diana and Topham's marriage was a happy one, despite his developing a fondness for laudanum (opium dissolved in alcohol); at the height of his addiction, he was taking up to 400 drops a day. Unfortunately, despite his acute sense of style, Beauclerk allowed himself to become increasingly dishevelled, and on one visit to Blenheim Palace the bewigged dandy boasted that he had enough lice about his person to people a parish!

One can only speculate about the good use to which scalp scratchers were put by the rest of the house guests when he visited: a most unfortunate state of affairs at a time when the fantastic hair creations of the period could stay in place for several days or weeks and were notoriously difficult to keep clean and vermin free.

CHAPTER 3

'Honi soit qui mal y pense'

'Evil be to he who evil thinks'

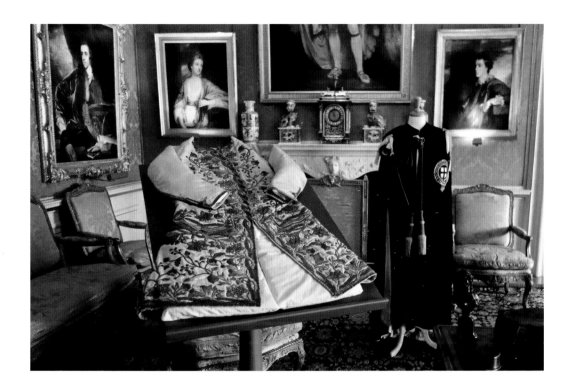

The Order of the Garter is the highest and oldest order of chivalry in England. It was founded in 1348 by King Edward III supposedly following a Court ball where a lady – Joan, Countess of Salisbury – lost one of her garters. In order to spare her blushes, the king bent down, picked it up and tied it around his own leg, promising that he would turn it into the most honoured garter ever worn and that the Order would be awarded to only the most worthy of his subjects.

The king's reprimand to the gathered assembly, 'honi soit qui mal y pense', became the motto of this honour and translates as 'evil be to he who evil thinks'. Originally, members of the Order were chosen only from the aristocracy, but today even commoners – and indeed women – can become a Knight or Lady

Companion of the Garter. It remains a very exclusive order, however, and its members are limited to HM Queen Elizabeth II at its head, a number of senior royals – including HRH The Prince of Wales and HRH The Duke of Cambridge – and then a further twenty-four non-royal Knights.

Many of the Dukes of Marlborough have held this particular honour, and the Green Drawing Room at Blenheim is dominated by George Romney's portrait of the 4th Duke of Marlborough (1739–1817) in his Garter robes. The robes themselves have not really changed in the hundreds of years since the Order was established. The Knights still wear a dark blue cloak fastened at the neck with blue and gold rope and a broad-brimmed hat with a low crown, decorated with a plume of ostrich

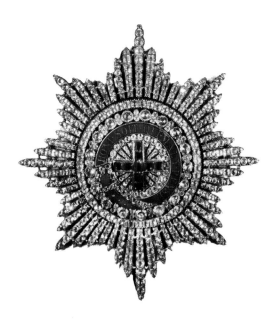

Previous page
Clothes denoted wealth
and social standing. There
were very strict rules
regarding what should be
worn on formal occasions
– particularly at court – and
woe betide anyone who
chose to ignore them.

left
A Garter star: part of the
Garter paraphernalia that
also includes a gold chain,
a garter and a broad-
brimmed hat topped with
ostrich feathers.

Below left
Portrait of George Spencer,
4th Duke of Marlborough,
by George Romney,
mid-1700s. Garter robes
are not exactly a fashion
statement, but the clothes
the duke is wearing
beneath them certainly
are.

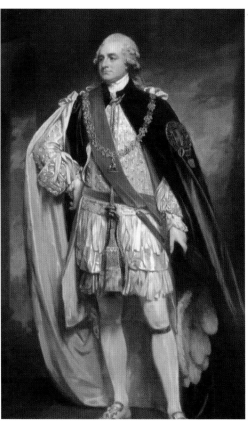

feathers. The duke (perhaps wisely) is shown holding his in his left hand.

It could be argued that Garter robes are not exactly a fashion statement, but the clothes the duke is wearing beneath them certainly are. Still, it seemed appropriate to include a set of robes in the display, but the most recent Duke of Marlborough to have been a Knight of the Garter was the 9th Duke (1871–1934), so I knew there was only a slim chance that we would still have his robes to display, assuming he had not hired them when needed. A little bit of sleuthing confirmed that this was indeed the case.

A little bit more sleuthing revealed that Ede & Ravenscroft, the gentlemen's outfitters established in 1689, was likely to have made the robes worn by the 4th Duke in his portrait. In fact, the robe rooms at Ede & Ravenscroft in Chancery Lane still make the majority of all ceremonial robes, as well as providing a storage facility for those nobles who own, rather than hire, such garments and do not have the space

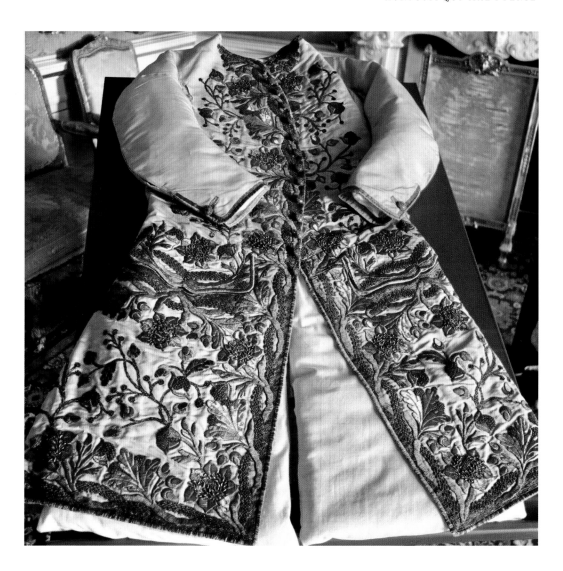

to store them. Thank heavens for Christopher Pickup! He and I first met when I was working on our 2016 exhibition commemorating 300 years since the birth of landscape architect, Lancelot 'Capability' Brown. The 4th Duke had been the one to commission Capability Brown to alter the landscape at Blenheim, so he had earned a place in that particular display, and now Chris came up trumps yet again, with the loan of the same set of Garter robes that

Above

It was very much de rigueur for men to wear court coats for formal occasions. It would not have been unusual for someone of the duke's rank and social standing to have hundreds of these beautiful items in his wardrobe. If he had worn the same one on more than a couple of occasions, it would have been commented upon and assumptions made about his financial status.

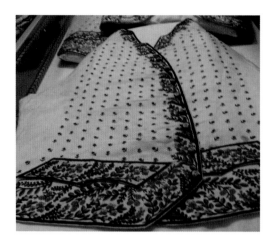

Left
A richly decorated
waistcoat would have been
worn beneath the court
coat.

Right
The court coats on display
in the Green Drawing
Room were made of the
finest silk and embroidered
with silk thread and also
threads of gold and silver.

had been on display to represent the duke the previous year.

At the court of King George III, a contemporary and friend of the 4th Duke, clothes continued to denote wealth and social standing. There were strict rules regarding what should be worn on formal occasions – particularly at court – and woe betide anyone who chose to ignore them. Technically, anyone could attend court events, as it was assumed that only the upper echelons of society would be able to afford the cost of the clothes required. There was a loophole, however. It was often the case that a nobleman or woman would leave items of clothing to a favourite servant: Sarah, the 1st Duchess of Marlborough, famously left half of her clothes (and £16,000, among other things) to her loyal maid, Grace Ridley.

When this occurred, a person from the lower orders would technically have the opportunity to be correctly dressed and thus be able to visit court along with his/her betters. If an individual was discovered to be wearing clothes above their station, however, then he or she would be ridiculed or even subjected to

violence for not having had the sense to have them altered appropriately. There was no danger of social mobility here.

It was very much de rigueur for men to wear court coats for formal occasions. A richly decorated waistcoat would have been worn beneath the court coat and it would not have been unusual for someone of the duke's rank and social standing to have hundreds of these beautiful items in his wardrobe. If he had worn the same one on more than a couple of occasions, it would have been commented upon and negative assumptions made about his financial status.

Sadly, none of the 4th Duke's clothing survives in the Blenheim collection: Althea to the rescue once more! The two court coats pictured were loaned to us and illustrate beautifully how the decoration on the coats became increasingly sophisticated and gave rise to exquisite examples of embroidery, particularly around pocket flaps and cuffs. Sometimes embroiderers would make use of the most unusual materials and it was not unheard of for shimmering fish scales to be

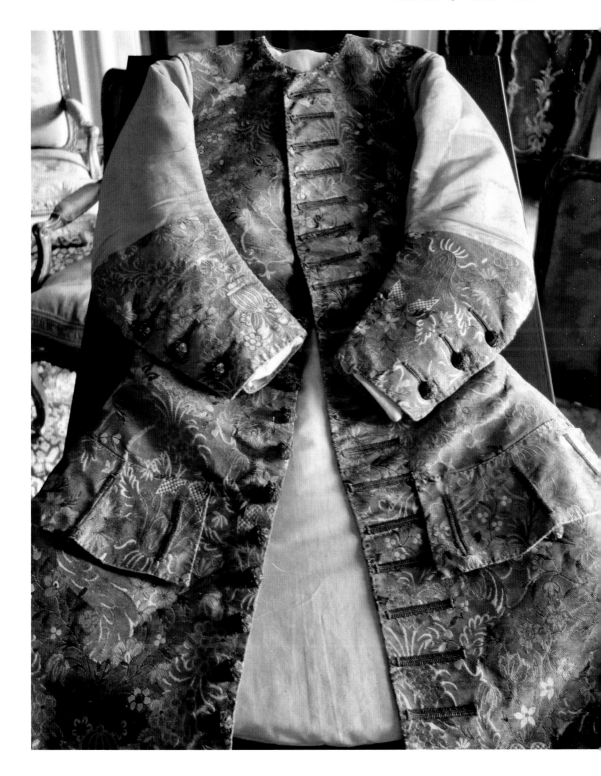

included to create a particular look. At times, men's clothes were so elaborate that women looked almost dowdy by comparison.

The court coats on display in the Green Drawing Room were made of the finest silk and embroidered with silk thread and also threads of gold and silver. Sequins were also used extensively in the decoration. Unlike the plastic ones of today, these were formed from silver wire, hammered and cut to form perfect circles. The effect by candlelight was stunning.

Although coats such as these could be afforded by only the wealthiest in society, the green court coat that we had on display was unusual: not only for its beauty, but also because, despite his obvious wealth, its owner thought to substitute the fabric at the top of the sleeves and the back with a plain, less expensive fabric in areas that would be covered by his

Ledger entries show that in 1704, the First Duke of Marlborough spent the equivalent of almost £0.5m on clothes in two months!

cloak and therefore remain unseen.

The 1st Duke of Marlborough was a constant presence at court from an early age and the cost of his suits and clothing grew at the same pace as his importance to Queen Anne. Ledger entries from 1704, the year of

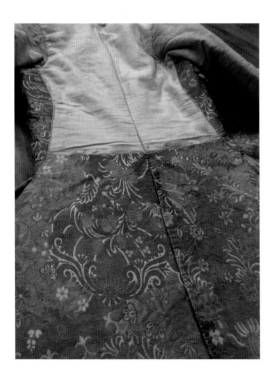

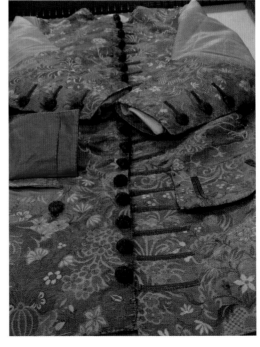

the Battle of Blenheim, list amounts totalling £2,069.16s.½d., which he spent on clothes from February to April that year. This is the equivalent of almost half a million pounds today and he thought nothing of paying £250 for just the buttons for a coat, but then they were probably made of silver.

It occurs to me at this point that no mention has been made of the role of garters in the Order of the Garter.

Both Knights and Ladies Companion still wear a garter as part of their regalia. Knights wear theirs buckled just below the left knee and Ladies Companion – to preserve decorum – wear theirs on the left arm. The garter worn by the men is typically blue velvet with gold embroidery around the edges and displays the motto of the Order of the Garter in gold lettering; gold roses are embroidered as stops between each word. The garter of Ladies Companion differs from the male version in that it is made of corded silk with heavy gold embroidery. These descriptions are fairly conservative, however, and in the past it was not unheard of for the wealthiest (or more ostentatious) holders of the honour to have the words of the motto picked out in diamonds.

Garters formed a staple part of the wardrobe of both men and women from as early as the fourteenth century, and until the advent of elastic they were tensioned by the use of tiny springs and fastened with buckles. The wearer would often have a message or rhyme sewn into the fabric of this relatively unprepossessing item and, although the surface area was tiny, it provided a further opportunity for embroidered decoration and enhancement, just in case anyone's eyes should fall upon it unexpectedly.

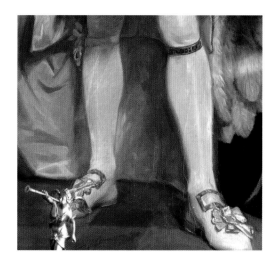

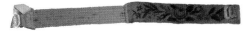

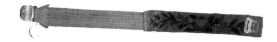

Far left
Coats such as these could be afforded by only the wealthiest in society. This example is unusual, not for its beauty but because, despite his obvious wealth, its wearer thought to substitute the fabric at the top of the sleeves and on the back with a plain, less expensive fabric in areas that would be covered by his cloak and therefore remain unseen.

Left
The pocket flaps are lined with a plain fabric to cut down on the cost of buying such an exquisite garment.

Above top
Detail from Portrait of George Spencer, 4th Duke of Marlborough, by George Romney, mid-1700s. Both Knights and Ladies Companion still wear a garter as part of their regalia. Knights wear theirs buckled just below the left knee and Ladies Companion – to preserve decorum – wear theirs on the left arm.

Above below
Garters formed a staple part of the wardrobe of both men and women from as early as the fourteenth century, and until the advent of elastic they were tensioned by the use of tiny springs and fastened with buckles.

33

CHAPTER 4

'Her eye-brows from a mouse's hide'

Excerpt from A Beautiful Young Nymph Going to Bed
by Jonathan Swift, 1731

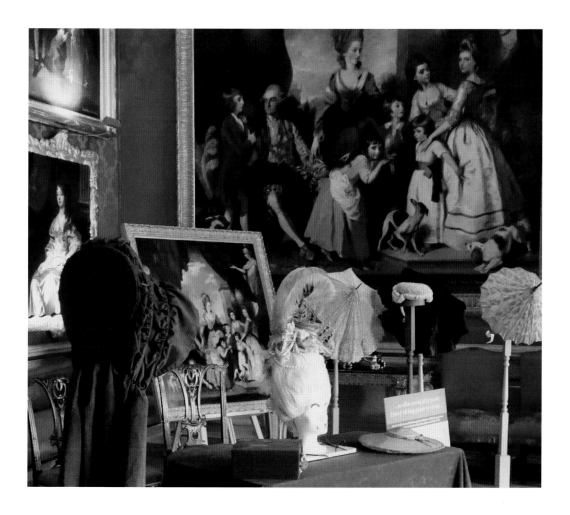

One of my favourite rooms in Blenheim Palace is the Red Drawing Room: not because of the proportions of the room itself, but rather because of what it contains. There are the quirky red, damask 'Chaperone Sofas', specially designed for surveillance and to keep budding young Victorian lovers at a respectable distance from each other; a hidden knife, which in case of fire can be used to cut the enormous canvases from their frames; and, at either end of the room, the two huge, full-length family portraits, one by John Singer Sargent of the 9th Duke and his family, and the other of the 4th Duke and his by Joshua Reynolds, a friend of the duke's sister, Lady Diana Beauclerk.

This latter portrait is truly superb, both for its fine workmanship and for the stories it tells and the characters it portrays.

It shows the duke – the Garter Knight we came across earlier – surrounded by six of his eight children. His wife Caroline Russell, a daughter of the Duke of Bedford, is pictured at the very centre of the painting where she

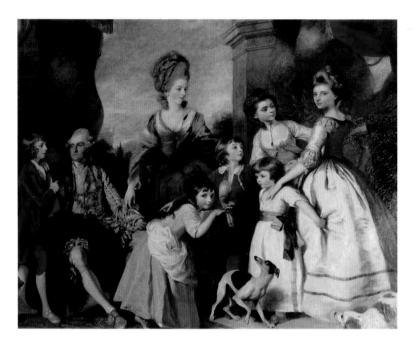

dominates the scene, just as she dominated
the life of her family. The 4th Duke's family
was the first of the Dukes of Marlborough to
use Blenheim Palace as a real home. It is easy
to imagine the long corridors ringing with
children's laughter and later, when the young
people acquired a taste for 'Theatricals', to
picture the vast Orangery converted to a
theatre complete with boxes that could seat
200 people.

Tickets for plays such as *The Deaf Lover* and
Cross Purposes were sent to 'persons of quality'
in and around Oxfordshire and the audience
was reminded to, 'laugh where you may, [but]
be candid where you can!' Apparently the
performances, whose casts included not only
family members, but also Oxford University
dons and students and, when absolutely
necessary, Blenheim servants, were sometimes
found to be lacking.

Caroline and the 4th Duke, who had been one
of the country's most eligible bachelors, were
married in 1762. Many aristocratic families
were related in some way or another and
they did their utmost to ensure that suitable
marriages – not necessarily love matches –
were made. Caroline's father was John Russell,
the 4th Duke of Bedford; his first wife, Lady
Diana Spencer, was the granddaughter of the
1st Duke and Duchess of Marlborough and
aunt to the 4th Duke. There was no blood
relationship between Lady Diana and Caroline
as Diana had died childless; Caroline's
mother was John Russell's second wife, the
Honourable Gertrude Leveson-Gower.

For hundreds of years the aristocracy were
the leaders of fashion: they could afford to be
and also had the advantage of access to the
latest trends in mainland Europe, particularly
France. Duchess Caroline was no exception

and she is pictured wearing a beautiful silk dress, her waist pinched in and one hand resting lightly on the duke's arm while she gazes, fondly perhaps, at her young family. The thing that really stands out when looking at this portrait is not naughty Charlotte, who teases her younger sister with a frightening mask, but rather the huge mass of hair that the duchess is balancing on her head. It is, of course, partly a wig.

The craze for wearing wigs – either a whole head or additional locks – first became popular in the seventeenth century. Like so many fashions it emerged from the French court and was soon adopted by the great and the good on this side of the Channel. When he was young, King Louis XIII liked to wear his hair long, but as it started to thin he made it appear more voluminous by the use of hairpieces and eventually full wigs. After a time, women also adopted the fashion and gradually the styles they favoured became increasingly outlandish, expensive and impractical. At one point during the period in which the wearing of wigs was de rigueur, it is said that Marie-Antoinette sported a 'head', as these hairpieces were

Once the Duchess' hair had been teased, curled and tonged into place it was covered in grease in preparation for the powder to be applied

known, that was at least 1 m high.

The Reynolds portrait is dated 1778: the period when wig-wearing literally reached the height of its popularity. The 'head' that Duchess Caroline is wearing would probably have been made from human hair rather than the less expensive horsehair, which many people had to settle for. It is unlikely to be a full wig, but rather her own hair combined with what today we would refer to as 'hair extensions'. The height and fullness were achieved by using a wire frame plus additional pads stuffed with wool or horsehair.

Once Caroline's hair had been teased, curled and tonged into place by an accomplished hairdresser, it was covered in a greasy paste made from bear grease, oil or fat, which served to stiffen the hair and to make it sticky. After this pomade had been used, the hair was ready to be coated in a perfumed powder, the all-important finishing touch. This was a slightly bizarre practice that took place in special 'powder rooms', where the powder was applied using a small set of bellows and different kinds of puffs: swansdown in the case of the Blenheim household, at a cost of 3s.6d. (17.5p) each. The wearer's clothes would be protected from the powder by a loose cape and the face by a cone-shaped mask that was held up against it and looked rather like a dunce's cap attached to a handle. It is unsurprising that the whole process of wig-wearing and dressing provided much fodder for the caricaturists of the day.

Just like the wigs themselves, the powder varied in quality from the coarsest produced from corn flour, to the best made from finely sieved starch. It was usually white – a colour that was thought to be most flattering – and violet was also a popular choice, as was

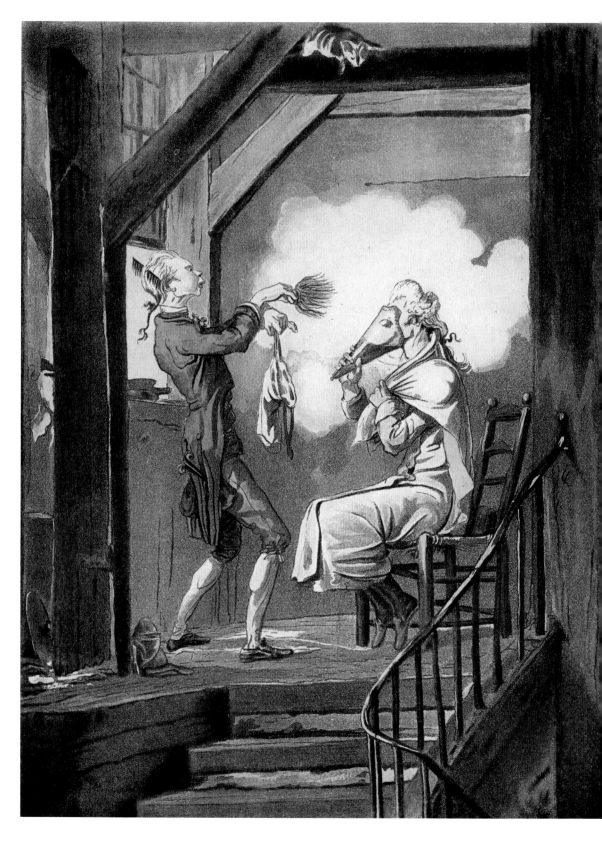

virtually every colour of the rainbow. The buyer would need to proceed with caution, however; genuine powder was not cheap and there were always unscrupulous merchants claiming to sell powder at below the market price. Unfortunately, this powder sometimes contained lime, chalk or even marble and would harm the hair and leave it in an even worse condition than was usual.

Although there were pamphlets written by hairdressers that described in detail how one could manage to dress one's own hair, these wondrous, skilful creations could not be achieved by a simple lady's maid or by the duchess herself. Caroline, like many of her peers, employed a French hairdresser. In her case it was a Monsieur Meseureur and he commanded an annual wage of £42, which was just a little less than the butler was paid (£45)

and more than twice the £20 the duke paid to his footmen. Meseureur would climb to the top of his portable wooden steps and, precariously balanced, carefully style the duchess's hair. When he was satisfied that his clay rollers and steel tongs had achieved the required curls, the hair would be powdered thoroughly and the look completed by the addition of decorations such as flowers and pearls, ribbons and feathers, and if the fancy took him, any number of ships in full sail.

This process would take many hours so, unsurprisingly, her hair, with its additional side curls, or 'favourites', and toupee (as the front portion was called), was dressed 'to keep' and the whole arrangement would stay put for weeks or even months at a time. This meant that when the duchess retired for the night, the adornments would be removed, and the hair

Left
Once a pomade had been added to the hair, it was ready to be covered in a perfumed powder, the all-important finishing touch. This was a slightly bizarre practice that took place in special 'powder rooms', as seen here in *The Toilet of an Attorney's Clerk*, by Antoine Charles Horace Vernet.

Right
Coiffeurs at work on an extravagant hairstyle: a contemporary satire on the fashionable excesses of the late eighteen century, c. 1774. The hairstylist would climb to the top of his portable wooden steps and, precariously balanced, carefully style the hair. When he was satisfied that his curling tongs had achieved the desired look, the hair would be powdered thoroughly and the whole thing decorated with flowers and pearls, ribbons and feathers, and if the fancy took him, any number of ships in full sail.

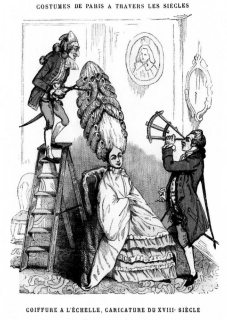

COSTUMES DE PARIS A TRAVERS LES SIÈCLES

COIFFURE A L'ÉCHELLE, CARICATURE DU XVIIIᵉ SIÈCLE

Nº 89.   (D'après une estampe du temps.)   F. Roy, éditeur.

Left

A bill from Monsieur Le Serré, the 1st Duke's wig-maker. It lists several different types of wig, but there is no mention of a Ramillies wig, which was named after the site of one of the duke's famous victories.

Above right

A range of wooden blocks used as a base in traditional wig-making.

Right

Handmade, bespoke, legal wigs are made using the same method employed over 300 years ago.

and extensions pinned into curls, ready to be combed out the following day, along with any loose or dirty powder and matted hair.

While she slept, Caroline's 'head' would be covered in a net – an early hairnet if you will – but considerably larger than those in use today. This served the dual purpose of helping to keep hairpins in, and trying to keep rodents and fleas out: the greasy paste that held the powder in place proved an attraction to many such creatures, so it was no wonder that a crucial part of a lady's accessories should be a small scalp scratcher, designed to give maximum relief from itching. Goodness knows what sights would meet M. Meseureur's eyes when the duchess's head was eventually opened. Perhaps anecdotal reports of finding a nest of mice inside were not wholly without foundation.

While Duchess Caroline favoured weaving additional pieces of hair into her own hair to create a voluminous style, others, such as the 1st Duke of Marlborough, preferred

full-length wigs, or perukes, which could be removed at night and regularly sent away for delousing, cleaning and resetting without any great inconvenience to himself. As wigs were incredibly expensive, particularly those made of human hair rather than horsehair, they were often bequeathed to surviving family members rather than being discarded after the owner's death.

Among the papers of the 1st Duke is a bill from his wigmaker, Monsieur Le Serré. It lists several different types of wig, although disappointingly there is no mention of a Ramillies wig, which was curled at the sides with a long plait down the back and named after the site of one of the duke's famous victories. There are, however, long wigs (£25), side wigs (£16) and twisted wigs (£6.9s.), and the bill covers a three-year period from November 1707 to November 1710. It is amusing to read that payment was not received until 12 July 1712 – almost two years later – and instead of

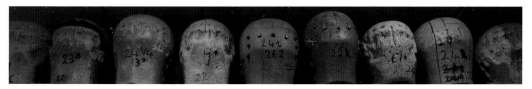

The greasy paste that held the powder in place proved an irresistible attraction to rodents and fleas

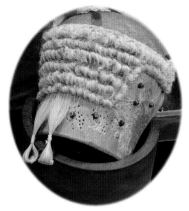

paying the total of £143.16s. in full, the duke allowed himself a discount of almost £12: certainly not for prompt payment!

In the eighteenth century just as today, the government was always quick to spot a money-making opportunity. Wigs were a prerogative of the wealthy, who could afford to be fashionable and, it was assumed, could afford to pay extra taxes. As a result of this, in 1786 Prime Minister William Pitt the Younger introduced a stamp duty on beauty preparations, which included hair powder, pomade, perfumes and even toothpaste. Ledger entries from 1787 relating to Duchess Caroline's expenditure typically show purchases of 'violet' or 'common powder' '& stamp'. Eventually, the duty became so prohibitively expensive that the wearing of wigs fell out of fashion and became the preserve of professions such as the legal profession and other figures of authority, or 'Big-Wigs' as they became known.

Few if any of these ancient wigs survive. Ede & Ravenscroft still produces handmade, bespoke legal wigs in Chancery Lane using exactly the same method it has employed for over 300 years. Having been fortunate enough to have had a tour of the robe and wig rooms, it would not surprise me to learn that the wooden blocks they use as a base when working on the wigs are the very ones used when the wig-making side of the business was first established by Thomas Ravenscroft in 1726. It is a fascinating process carried out by a small team of highly skilled wig-makers working with horsehair, who crimp and curl just as their predecessors did hundreds of years ago. Again, we were fortunate in being able to loan a wig that, although it is for use in the legal profession today, resembled perfectly the one worn by the 4th Duke in the portrait by Reynolds.

Acquiring an authentic eighteenth-century lady's wig proved to be problematic until we found a marvellous wig-maker, James Webber, who was able to produce a stupendous creation using traditional techniques. The result was a 45-cm-high wig, made from horsehair over a padded wire frame, adorned with pearls, ribbon, ostrich feathers and, as though that were not enough, three galleons in full sail. It was an absolute masterpiece.

The one thing I did not like quite so much about James's wig was the head upon which it had been made. It was white polystyrene and quite unattractive. All was not lost, however, and the face became a useful way of being able to illustrate the white complexion that, contrary to those of us today who aspire to a healthy looking tan, was the goal of both men

and women during the eighteenth century and earlier.

Exquisite lace or silk parasols were used to protect the face from the sun's harmful rays. These were attached to fine, decorative handles of cane or ivory and embellished with fur, feathers or tassels. The most interesting one that we had on display was a rather ingenious small, brown silk affair, which doubled as a riding crop. It would have been quite something to have seen that particular parasol in action.

Although parasols could be used to shade the face, the skin itself was actually whitened by applying concoctions containing harmful ingredients such as lead. Ceruse, a popular

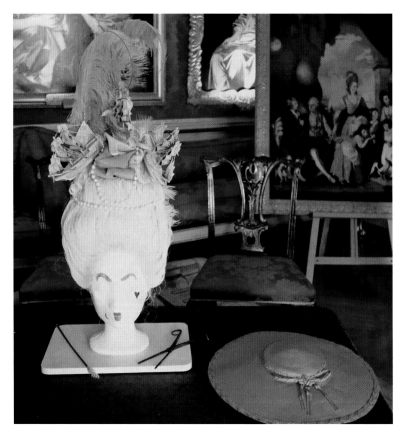

Left
A shallow-crowned straw bergère alongside a 45-cm-high wig, made in the traditional way from horsehair over a padded wire frame then adorned with pearls, ribbon, ostrich feathers and, as though that were not enough, three galleons in full sail. An absolute masterpiece!

Right
Exquisite lace or silk parasols were used to protect the face from the sun's harmful rays. These were attached to fine, decorative handles of cane or ivory and embellished with fur, feathers or tassels. Some of the most interesting ones were designed to double as a riding crop.

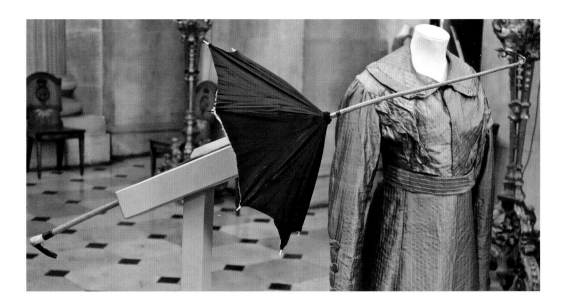

lead-based paste, was certainly effective in whitening the skin; unfortunately, it also caused tiredness, heart disease, gout, kidney failure and anaemia, teeth and hair loss, and, in extreme cases, death. Two notable beauties of the time who were said to be victims of this type of poisoning were the courtesan Kitty Fisher – she who found Lucy Locket's pocket in the nursery rhyme (see p. 106) – and the Irish beauty Maria Gunning, later Countess of Coventry, whose mother when casting around for suitably noble husbands for her daughters had had her mind very firmly set on a match between one of them and the future 5th Duke of Marlborough, once the little boy pictured in maroon velvet standing next to his father in the Reynolds' portrait.

The ingredients for some of the cosmetic preparations were not only bizarre by today's standards, but also rather costly and, like many things, the preserve of the rich. Poorer women tended to use herbal concoctions on their skin,

which ironically turned out to be a far safer option. There were various recipes to be had for almost any skin condition: for whitening the skin, for removing any hint of a tan and for disguising wrinkles, among others, which called for concoctions with ingredients such as tin, flour, rice, cuttlefish, calves' feet, pearls, whale fat and even nine-day-old puppies!

Once the ceruse had been applied, cheeks were rouged, lips were painted and black patches – or 'mouches' – were placed strategically on the face and breast. If you look carefully at the faces of Duchess Caroline and the mannequin, you will notice the beautifully rosy cheeks, which were less the outcome of healthy outdoor exercise and more the result of the application of an oil or paste to redden them: a type of rouge if you will. Again, the recipes for these pastes were numerous and could be almost as harmful as those used to whiten the complexion. A typical preparation would include ingredients such as a red-

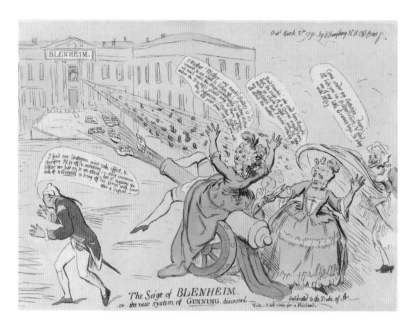

Mrs Gunning when casting around for suitably noble husbands for her daughters had once had her mind very firmly set on a match between one of them and the future 5th Duke of Marlborough and 'laid siege' on Blenheim Palace

Below right
Mice were unwelcome visitors in many households and in more extreme cases, they were trapped, skinned and the hide or tail cut, shaped and stuck on to replace missing eyebrows.

coloured extract from scaly cochineal bugs (still used to colour food like crab sticks), vinegar, brandy, red lead or mercury.

The patches were a useful part of a woman's toilet. As well as highlighting the whiteness of the wearer's skin, they would also serve to cover any disfiguring scars, typically those left behind by a dose of smallpox, syphilis or the effects of lead poisoning. The 'mouches' (French 'fly') were made from taffeta, paper, leather or silk and cut into various shapes – stars, moons, hearts or even a horse and carriage – and could be used to indicate mood, passion or political allegiance: an early version of the emoji, perhaps.

Members of the 1st Duchess's family and almost certainly Caroline herself used patches: entries in her ledgers show how many sheets of patches were purchased, as well as the tiny decorative boxes in which to store them. In 1706 four papers of patches cost the princely

sum of 2 shillings (10p, or just under £23 in 2017). This entry is on the same page as a payment of a little over double that amount for a Christmas tip to the 'Brewer's man and the Tallow Chandler's man', who were given 5 shillings each. The patches were as expensive as the Christmas tips were generous.

Once make-up and patches were in place, attention could be turned to the eyebrows. If these had not already fallen out as a result of lead poisoning, they would be shaved off and high, thin brows would be drawn in using lead or burnt cork, or replaced with false ones made from mouse skins, giving the wearer a look of perpetual surprise. Mice were unwelcome visitors in many households and in more extreme cases they were trapped, skinned and the hide or tail cut, shaped and stuck onto the lady's face. For the exhibition, the Blenheim carpenters came up trumps: not in supplying mice, but in making a replica mousetrap. Their help and cooperation in creating this, along with their splendid work in making stands for many of the trickier items for display – hats, shoes, aprons, coats – was invaluable.

It is of course interesting to look at historic perceptions of beauty and understandable that we should express surprise or revulsion at the methods used. I am sure that in years to come future generations will be just as amazed at the popularity of certain types of cosmetic surgery and the fake tanning that is popular today, not to mention the fillers used to gain a face that does not age, or which does not even move in the case of Botox and other facial procedures.

Satirist Jonathan Swift (1667–1745) had very cynical views about what was going on with the toilet habits of the eighteenth-century woman and the artifice employed to appear fashionable. One of his most famous works dates back to 1731 and describes in nauseating detail the bedtime routine of Corinna, a woman of the night:

...seated on a three-legged chair,
Takes off her artificial hair:
Now, picking out a crystal eye,
She wipes it clean, and lays it by.
Her eye-brows from a mouse's hide,
Stuck on with art on either side,

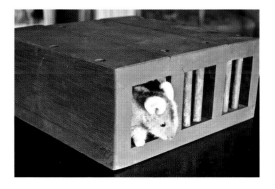

He goes on to describe her removing the stays and padding that artificially shape her body before she turns to the job of removing her ceruse and rouge:

But must, before she goes to bed,
Rub off the dawbs of white and red;

The following morning, Corinna must first deal with the ravages of the night before reapplying her camouflage:

...Shock her tresses filled with fleas.
The nymph, tho' in this mangled plight,
Must ev'ry morn her limbs unite.
But how shall I describe her arts
To recollect the scattered parts?
Or shew the anguish, toil, and pain,
Of gath'ring up herself again?

Excerpts from *'A Beautiful Young Nymph Going to Bed'* (1731) by Jonathan Swift.

Although Swift, author of *Gulliver's Travels* (1726), exaggerates the case somewhat, there was at that time a school of thought who feared that heavily made-up women would be able to dupe wealthy, unsuspecting bachelors into marriage. This practice was regarded as being akin to witchcraft and in 1770 an amendment was proposed to the Witchcraft Act. Its aim was to protect men from being tricked into marriage by the use of padding and false adornments that included, among other things, perfume, cosmetics, false teeth or hairpieces. It is interesting to note that, not without reason, the Italian word for 'make-up' is 'trucco', or 'trick'.

CHAPTER 5

'Hats, remarkable large'

'Hats, remarkable large: some as large as… round breakfast tables'

A description of hats, The Gentleman's and London Magazine, *1777*

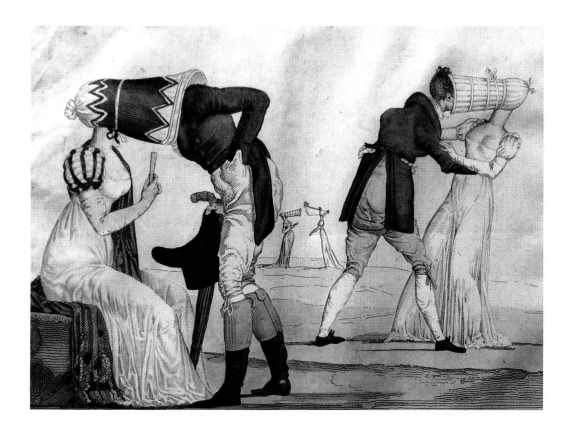

The relationship between Queen Anne and Sarah, the 1st Duchess of Marlborough, is well documented, as is the fact that the queen was incredibly generous in gifting the Manor of Woodstock to John Churchill, as well as £240,000 with which to build himself a palace. Given this, it seemed appropriate to display here a rare example of a split cane hat that once belonged to Sarah's childhood friend. It was designed to look like reticella, a type of Venetian cutwork lace popular from the Medieval period. These straw/cane hats were a favourite with Anne's ladies at court, but hats in the form that we understand them today did not become really popular until the mid-1700s and replaced earlier headdresses.

Let us return for a moment to the question of a lady's hair. As 'heads' grew higher and changed shape, so the hat-maker adapted styles to accommodate them. I use the term 'hat-maker' advisedly, as during the eighteenth century milliners dealt with the supply and creation of trimmings and adornments required for the hat, rather than with the actual process of hat-making. It was not until the nineteenth century that the term 'milliner' was used to describe a maker of hats and trimmings.

In the famous painting by Thomas Gainsborough, Georgiana, Duchess of Devonshire, a cousin of the 4th Duke of

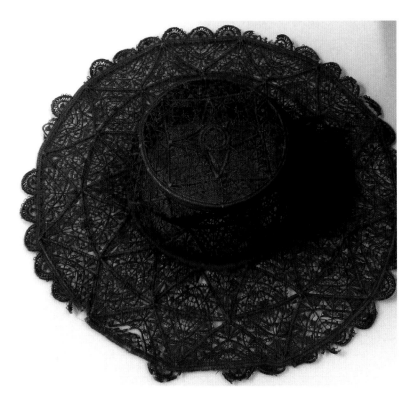

Previous page
Caricatures Parisiennes:
*Les Invisibles en Tête-à-
Tête*, published by Aaron
Martinet, late 1810s.
This French cartoon is
lampooning poke bonnets
so large that the wearer
could keep all but the most
determined at bay.

Left
A rare example of a
split cane hat that once
belonged to Queen Anne.
It was designed to look like
reticella, a type of Venetian
cutwork lace.

Marlborough, is seen wearing an enormous wide-brimmed picture hat with a deep crown. It could easily be likened to a breakfast table in both size and shape. It is decorated with ribbon and ostrich feathers and sits atop her huge powdered hair with frizzed (back-combed) sides and long hairpieces. This type of hat was one response to the big hair of the day; the simple shallow-crowned 'bergère' was another. Essentially a straw hat, it would be perched carefully on top of a lady's hair and set at a jaunty angle for best effect.

In inclement weather ladies would wear a calash in addition to their hat. Named after the seventeenth-century carriage that bore the same name, the calash grew in size as hairstyles did and looked just like the hood of a pram. The hood was attached to a cape and was made of lined, weather-proofed silk, taffeta or cotton, then stretched over half hoops of cane. This meant that the hood stood proud from the hair and was less likely to spoil the fruits of the hairdresser's labour. The one we had on display in the Red Drawing Room looked rather sinister with its dark empty interior and reminded me of the fearsome 'Dementors' that inhabit the world of Harry Potter.

Over a hundred years after the death of Queen Anne (and a succession of Georges and one William), Great Britain saw the coronation of a petite but powerful queen. Queen Victoria was until recently our longest-serving monarch and her reign saw many changes and developments: not only in industry but

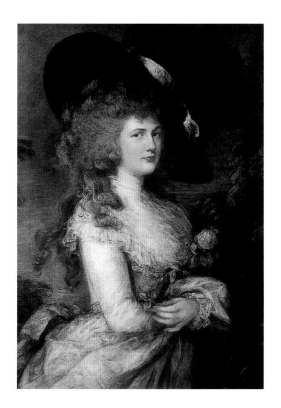

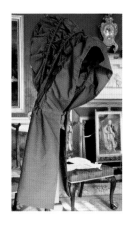

Left
Detail from *Portrait of Georgiana, Duchess of Devonshire*, by Thomas Gainsborough, 1785–87. A cousin of the 4th Duke of Marlborough, Georgiana is wearing an enormous wide-brimmed picture hat with a deep crown. It resembles a breakfast table both in size and shape. Decorated with ribbon and ostrich feathers, it sits atop her huge powdered hair with its frizzed sides and long hairpieces.

Below
As hair reached greater heights, one response was the bergère: a shallow-crowned straw hat that would be perched carefully on top of a lady's hair and set at a jaunty angle for best effect.

Above
In inclement weather, ladies would wear a calash in addition to their hat. Named after the seventeenth-century carriage that bore the same name, the calash grew in size as hairstyles did and looked just like the hood of a pram.

also, inevitably, in fashion. Staying with the theme of heads and hats, wigs and large hair became unfashionable, even at court, and soon women were following the queen's example and parting their hair in the centre, drawing most of it up into a bun but allowing a cluster of side curls, ringlets or plaits to add interest in front of the ears. Hats were again required to accommodate the change in hairstyles and women took to wearing the bonnet outdoors and a simple cap indoors. In fact, other than for riding, when a top hat might be worn, a variation on the bonnet was considered to be the correct type of headwear for all occasions.

The shape of the bonnet changed throughout the Victorian period. It was stiffened and made from either straw, velvet, horsehair or

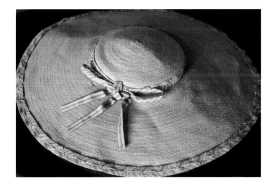

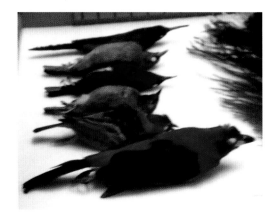

felt. Brims became bigger, then smaller; they were an integral part of the whole or formed a straight line with the crown. Trimmings also varied tremendously. Silk ribbon was popular as were satin, lace, artificial flowers and, rather controversially both then and now, taxidermied birds, including tiny hummingbirds with their much sought-after beautiful, colourful plumage. The 'Wearing of Feathers' elicited a heated correspondence in The Times in the autumn of 1893 and called for women to unite to 'control the vagaries and cruelties of those fashions of which...they [were] the unresisting slaves'.

Men too continued to wear hats during this

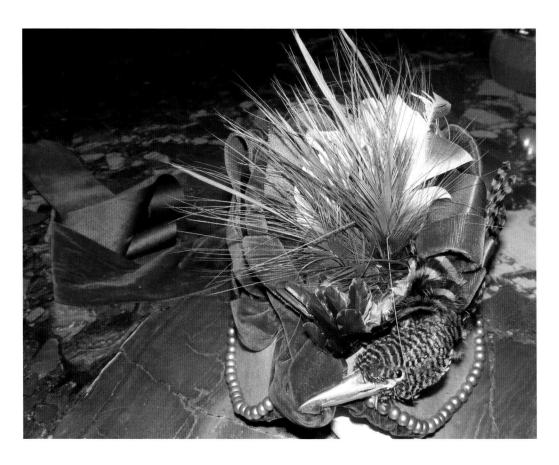

era. Top hats made from felted beaver fur were popular, and for indoor use a smoking cap, decoratively embroidered and often enhanced with a tassel or two. It was considered extremely improper for women to smoke at this time and so it was out of consideration for the so-called fairer, weaker sex that gentlemen covered their heads while indulging in this habit, in a room kept especially for this purpose, thus protecting their ladies from the all-pervading smell of tobacco emanating from their hair.

Blenheim Palace has a special and rather long-standing relationship with the House of Dior – more of which later – so it seemed especially meaningful to bring a contemporary hat into the small collection on display. Enter the marvellous Stephen Jones, who in 2016 celebrated twenty years of designing and making hats for Dior, working firstly alongside head designer John Galliano and then subsequent creative directors right up to and including Maria Grazia Chiuri, who took the helm in 2016.

Stephen graduated from St Martin's School of Art and early on in his career he created hats for Boy George, Steve Strange and Diana, Princess of Wales, among others. He remains an inspiration to blossoming young milliners and his creations feature regularly on the covers of *Vogue* and *Harper's Bazaar*. Stephen famously 'hatted' Doria Ragland, mother of Meghan Markle, HRH The Duchess of Sussex, on the occasion of her marriage to HRH The Duke of Sussex in May 2018.

The term 'hat' when used in connection with Stephen Jones is insubstantial and misleading. Yes, Stephen's creations tend to be worn on (or around) the head, but his imagination knows

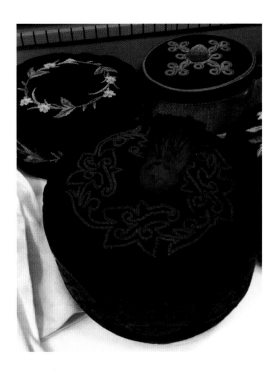

Top left
Trimmings for bonnets varied tremendously. Silk ribbon was popular as were satin, lace, artificial flowers and, controversially, taxidermied birds, including tiny hummingbirds with their much sought-after colourful plumage.

Left
A small bonnet trimmed with ribbon, a taxidermied bird and pearls.

Above
Men wore smoking caps indoors. It was considered extremely improper for women to smoke during this period, so out of consideration for the so-called fairer, weaker sex gentlemen covered their heads while indulging in this habit. In this way, ladies were protected from the all-pervading smell of tobacco that would otherwise emanate from a gentleman's hair.

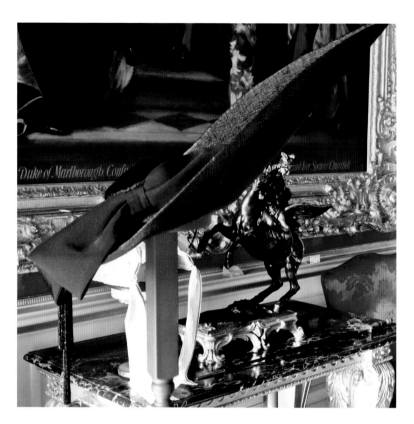

no bounds and, if the occasion demands it, you could end up sporting a paint palette, a giant cotton reel or what appears to be a flimsy lace mask and still be able to claim that you are wearing a hat.

When I contacted his office to see if he would be willing to let us exhibit an item from his considerable archive, Stephen and his Press and Communications Manager, Annika Lievesley, could not have been more helpful. I was sent a number of images and asked to select a hat. Sheer bliss!

I alighted upon a large, tasselled, black straw creation that happened to be called 'The Favourite'. It turned out that it had been inspired by the fabulous black and white

hat worn by Audrey Hepburn at Ascot in the 1965 film, *My Fair Lady*. It looked very much at home in its palatial surroundings, once it had been carefully displayed on its specially made hat stand. When Stephen Jones came to Blenheim to address a sell-out audience in the Long Library, I had the opportunity to chat to him about it.

Stephen told me that in 2009 he had curated the Victoria and Albert Museum's first ever hat exhibition. During the period leading up to it, he managed to track down a number of iconic hats and among them, stuffed at the bottom of a huge box in a Warner Brothers store room in Los Angeles, he discovered the very hat that had been the inspiration for his own. It

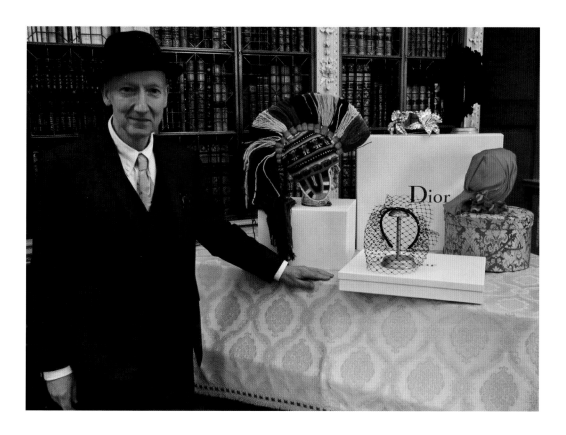

Blenheim Palace has a special relationship with the House of Dior so it seemed appropriate to bring a hat by Stephen Jones into the small collection on display

will perhaps come as no surprise to learn that one of the eight Oscars awarded to the film went to society favourite Cecil Beaton for best costumes, which of course included the hat.

For Stephen, finding Audrey Hepburn's battered hat must have been like finding the Holy Grail. After much negotiation, it was agreed that in return for restoring it to its former glory, Stephen would be allowed to display this amazing find for a short period during his V&A exhibition, and his career continues to go from strength to strength.

Not bad for a young man whose first attempt at hat-making incorporated a spray of plastic flowers that his mother had got free many years earlier with a well-known brand of petrol!

CHAPTER 6

Liveries and lace

Military uniforms and servant liveries were based on the fashions of the day

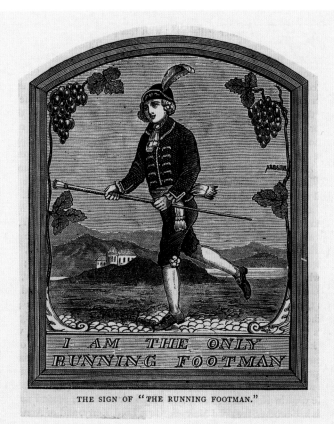

THE SIGN OF "THE RUNNING FOOTMAN."

The Green Writing Room at Blenheim Palace houses one of the most glorious items in its collection: the Blenheim Tapestry. For those of you who may have wondered how the Palace came to be built, the answer is simply this: it was built because of the Battle of Blenheim.

I have lived in Oxfordshire since the early 1980s and, to my embarrassment, the first time I set foot in Blenheim Palace was when I went along for a job interview in 2008. Even more embarrassing was the fact that I thought that the battlefields of Blenheim must be somewhere in Oxfordshire or one of the adjacent counties, thinking along the lines of the famous battles of Edgehill and Naseby. Blenheim (or Blindheim as it should correctly be called) is in fact in Bavaria, about 120 km from Munich and many more from Blenheim Palace.

The Battle of Blenheim was a key in the War of the Spanish Succession, in which French troops were defeated by the 1st Duke of Marlborough on 13 August 1704. It was a turning point in English history and Queen Anne thought it appropriate to further reward John Churchill, her most able of generals. She had already given him a dukedom and

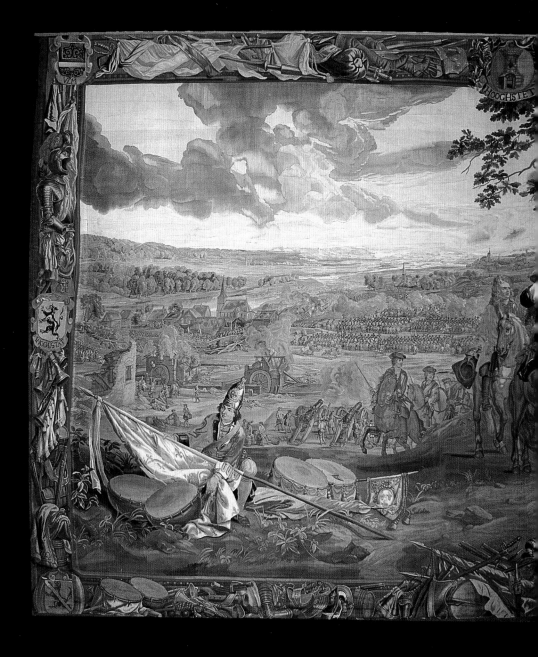

Above

The Blenheim Tapestry was woven in the Flemish workshop of Judocus de Vos over a period of many years and designed by Philippe de Hondt from maps and sketches provided by the 1st Duke. It is an amazing feat of craftsmanship.

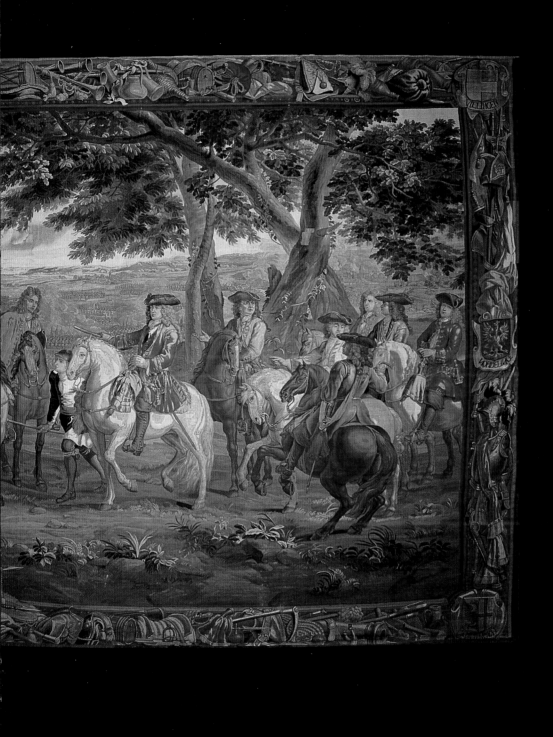

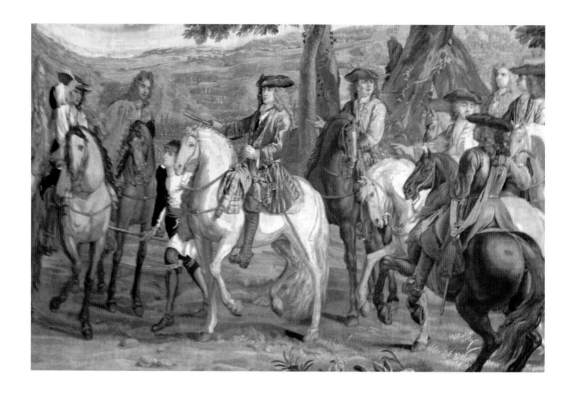

plied him and his ambitious wife, Sarah, with riches and power, so now she decided to make him a gift of around 800 hectares of land and a crumbling manor house in which Princess Elizabeth, the future Queen Elizabeth I, had once been imprisoned.

As though this were not enough, Queen Anne also gave John Churchill the sum of £240,000 from the public purse. This was not only to express the nation's gratitude in delivering it from the enemy, but also to give the duke the necessary funds to build Blenheim: it was almost enough to build a palace, but not quite, and the Duke had to add a further £60,000 from his own pocket to complete the building. As you can imagine, this equates to many millions today, so it may be taken as read that Queen Anne was very

pleased with her loyal servant.

The Blenheim Tapestry is an amazing piece of craftsmanship. It was woven in the Flemish workshop of Judocus de Vos over a period of many years and designed by Philippe de Hondt from maps and sketches provided by the 1st Duke. It depicts rows of soldiers ranked alongside the River Danube and the tiny village of Blindheim, from which the word 'Blenheim' is derived, can be seen in the background. Central to all of this is the 1st Duke himself, baton of office in hand, taking the surrender of Marshal Tallard, the head of the defeated French army. In the bottom left-hand corner, a Grenadier Guard is seen taking possession of the standard of the defeated French forces, symbolising their utter defeat.

One of the most striking things about the

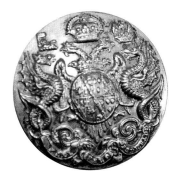

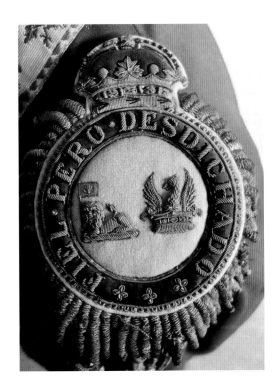

Left
Detail from *The Blenheim Tapestry*. Before national armies were established, small, private armies were raised and funded by wealthy and powerful men. The colour and style of the military uniforms tended to resemble the liveries worn by their household servants.

Above & right
The monogrammed gold braid was referred to as 'lace'. The liveries would incorporate the family coat of arms or monogram, typically on the epaulettes and the solid silver buttons of the coat or jacket.

tapestry is the level of detail, especially of the soldiers' uniforms. Before national armies were established, small, private armies were raised and funded by wealthy and powerful men, and the colour and style of the military uniforms tended to resemble the liveries worn by their household servants. That being the case, it is no wonder that the word livery is used to describe both the uniform worn by the common soldier and also that worn by senior male servants in an aristocratic household such as this: the implication being that the wearer belonged to, or depended upon, the person who supplied it.

Military uniforms and servant liveries were based on the fashionable styles of the day and, as with military uniforms that have regular combat uniform as well as dress uniform, a servant would have plain livery for when just the family was in residence – or indeed when they were at other residences – and 'laced' livery for formal occasions. The 'lace' was in fact monogrammed gold braid. The liveries would also incorporate the family coat of arms or monogram, typically on the epaulettes and the solid silver buttons of the coat or jacket. All these decorations and enhancements meant that the identity of the master of the household was left in no doubt and neither was his social and financial standing, nor the status of an occasion: a visit from royalty perhaps. The grander the occasion, the grander and more highly decorated the livery.

Clothing a regiment of servants was quite an expense: senior male members of staff had to be provided with jackets, coats, breeches,

This page
Illustration by an unknown artist of Christian Davies (also known as Kit Cavanagh), who fought at both the Battle of Schellenberg and at the Battle of Blenheim while searching for her errant husband. She was the first female Chelsea Pensioner.

Right
In the account ledgers the running footman's uniform is listed separately from other Blenheim liveries: he wore a 'crimson cloth frock, a buff cloth waistcoat and a pair of crimson shag breeches' as well as a 'petticoat and sash' all for the princely sum of £9.6s.0d.

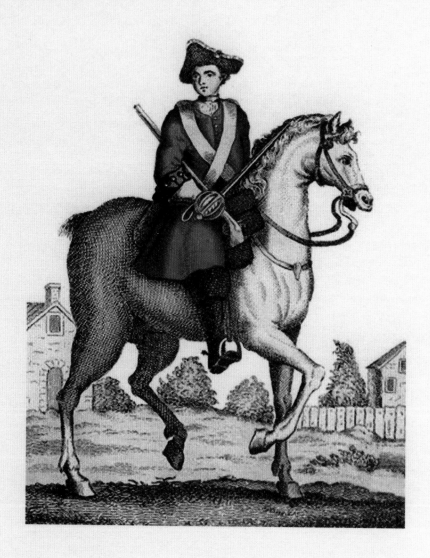

waistcoats, shoes, stockings and hats. Perhaps it was just as well that underwear as we know it today had yet to put in an appearance! A look at the Blenheim ledgers shows that vast amounts of money were spent clothing the staff. For example, in the early 1700s a plain livery for a footman cost £5.14s.4½d. (£5.72), the equivalent of £972 today.* It is incredible to think that this was almost as much as his annual wage of £6. It is no wonder that liveries were designed to last for years and passed down from servant to servant.

An additional expense was that the duke and duchess had several houses. Not all of the servants would travel with them when they visited their various homes, so uniforms had to be provided for many servants in several establishments.

It was not unheard of for a Duke of Marlborough to employ servants to fulfil more unusual roles, such as dressing blisters, cleaning teeth or running ahead of his coach in the case of a running footman. The running footman was always to be found in close proximity to the duke and accordingly his livery far outshone even the grandeur of that of his peers. He was extremely useful not only in heralding his master's arrival but also, given his grand physique, in preventing the coach from toppling over on sharp bends.

A ledger entry for 15 April 1709 shows the livery for the running footman listed separately from other Blenheim liveries: he wore a 'crimson cloth frock, a buff cloth waistcoat and a pair of crimson shag breeches' as well as a 'petticoat and sash' all for the princely sum of £9.6s.0d. (£9.30), the equivalent of around £1,500 today.*

Various names appear in the Blenheim

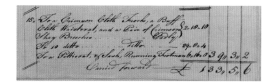

ledgers as holders of this exalted position, which commanded an annual wage of £20. Sadly, towards the end of the eighteenth century a running footman expired after competing in a race from London to Windsor, against the duke's horse-drawn coach. A distance of 96 km at an average speed of 11 km per hour was just too much, even when buoyed up by regular sips of brandy and egg from a silver container at the top of the staff he carried as he ran.

No further reference is made to this particular post in the household staff after this sad occurrence.

Although liveries – military or civilian – were worn only by men, in the early eighteenth century, unbeknown to the 1st Duke of Marlborough, there was a woman in his army who proudly wore the livery of the Scots Greys regiment. She actually fought at both the Battle of Schellenberg and at the Battle of Blenheim while she searched for her errant husband. The story of Christian Davies (1667–1739), also known as Kit Cavanagh, is one filled with excitement, bravery and danger. She eventually found her husband in the arms of another woman and so decided to continue with her life as a soldier.

Christian Davies was wounded at the Battle of Ramilles in 1706, and it was at this point that her true identity as a woman was revealed and she was no longer allowed to fight. However, her

*Bank of England inflation calculator

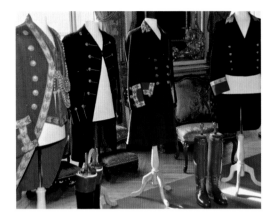

It was considered inappropriate for women to wait at the Duke's table until the 1980s

actions did not go unrewarded: Queen Anne was so impressed with Davies's actions that she awarded her a payment of £50 and a lifetime pension of 1 shilling (5p) a day. Davies retired to the Royal Hospital Chelsea where she lived until her death in 1739. She is buried alongside other retired soldiers in the burial ground in the Royal Hospital grounds.

After his marriage to American heiress Consuelo Vanderbilt in 1895, the 9th Duke of Marlborough was able to spend money on the much-needed upkeep of the Palace. He was also in a position to show the rest of the world that he was now a man of financial substance. Like many of the Marlborough dukes before him, he required his most senior and most visible male servants to be appropriately dressed in the Marlborough livery; the lesser ranks were dressed in morning suits of the type that most servants wore at that time.

The liveries pictured in this book date back to the late 1890s and were designed to resemble those worn by Blenheim servants in the eighteenth century. They were worn by the 'front of house' staff: the footmen, coachmen and gatemen of the 9th Duke. Of all of them, the footman's uniform of maroon breeches, braided jacket, silk stockings and black patent leather buckled shoes is perhaps the most impressive.

The 9th Duke, who was of a rather diminutive stature, employed only footmen who were at least 182 cm tall. Presumably having footmen of a uniform size also helped when it came to recycling the clothing. With the duke's insistence on their continuing the eighteenth-century fashion for powdering their hair, these statuesque footmen cut rather a dash.

Mrs Ryman, the 9th Duke's housekeeper and most senior member of his female staff, was just required to wear a smart, dark frock; there are few – if any – references in the ledgers to expenditure for the clothing of female staff. In his 1945 account of life below stairs, former Hall Boy Gerald 'Johnny' Horner notes that the female servants were actually supplied with a plain black dress to wear when carrying out their daily tasks; he remarks that this was relatively unusual. The female servants were very much 'back of house' and did not warrant such splendid uniforms. In fact, in this household it was not considered appropriate for female staff to wait at the duke's table until the 1980s.

Left

These liveries date back to the late 1890s and were designed to resemble those worn by Blenheim servants in the eighteenth century. They were worn by the 'front of house' staff: the footmen, coachmen and gatemen of the 9th Duke.

Right

After his marriage to American heiress Consuelo Vanderbilt who brought with her a sizeable dowry, the 9th Duke of Marlborough was able to ensure that his male servants were appropriately dressed in the Marlborough livery. Even the backs of the liveries worn by his most senior and most visible staff were as ornate and as expensively adorned as the fronts.

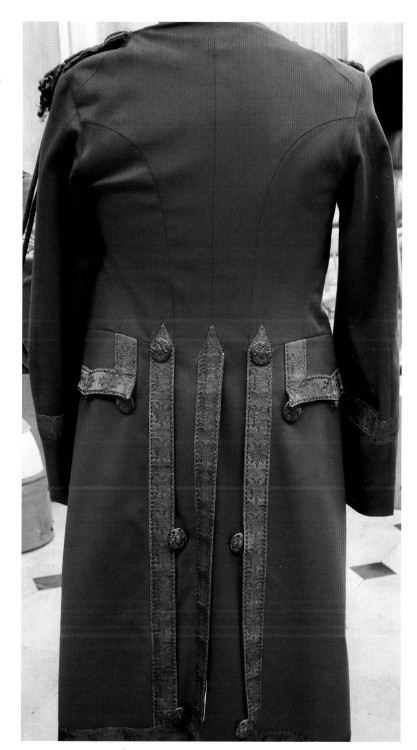

CHAPTER 7

'I like to look tidy and neat'

'I like to look tidy and neat,
not... loose and négligé'

From an 1889 discussion on corsets

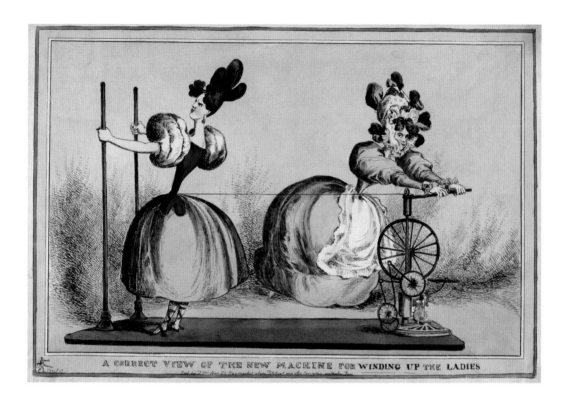

A CORRECT VIEW OF THE NEW MACHINE FOR **WINDING UP THE LADIES**

Richard Buckner's portrait of Churchill's beloved grandmother, Frances, the 7th Duchess of Marlborough (1822–1899), shows her dressed according to the fashion of the time. She is tightly corseted and the skirt of her dress is covered in frills, flounces and furbelows. In contrast, the 1928 portrait of Mary, the 10th Duchess of Marlborough (1900–1961), shows a slim, elegant figure with short Marcel-waved hair, dressed in a loose-fitting ankle-length evening dress. Despite there being only seventy years or so between the portraits, the two duchesses could not be further apart in terms of what they are wearing, and this applies to both underwear and outerwear.

Frances's meringue of a dress is fashioned from many metres of fabric, while Mary's dress could easily be cut from just a few. Mary's dress is unadorned; Frances's is just the opposite. Both the duchesses are wearing pearls: Mary's are limited to a single strand at her throat, while Frances's can be seen at her neck, ear lobes and bosom and even sewn into the bodice of her dress.

It is interesting to note that today it would pass completely unremarked if one were to wear the dress Mary is wearing in her 1928 portrait. It would have been most remarkable, however, for Mary to have worn the dress seen in Frances's picture, despite the fact that roughly the same period of time had elapsed between the painting of Frances's and Mary's portraits, and from the date of Mary's portrait and today. In fact, genuine vintage clothes are currently treasured and worn with pride, while

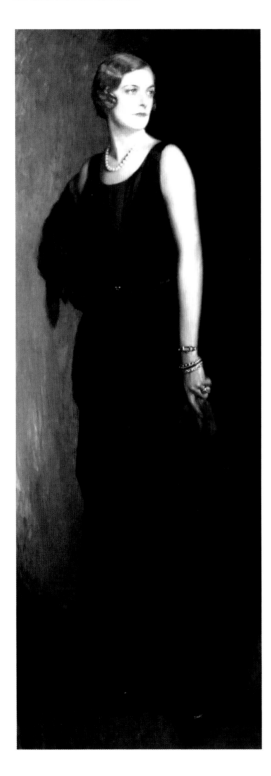

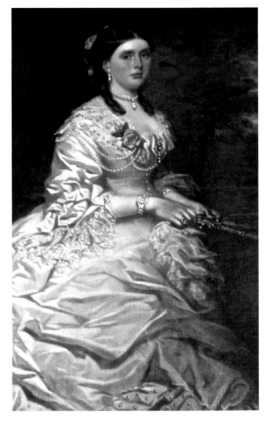

Previous page
*A Correct View of the New
Machine for Winding Up
the Ladies,* by Thomas
McLean, published c. 1830.

Above
*Frances, 7th Duchess of
Marlborough,* by Richard
Buckner, mid-1800s.
Dressed according to
the fashion of the time,
Frances is tightly corseted
and her skirt is covered
in frills, flounces and
furbelows.

Left
*Mary, 10th Duchess of
Marlborough,* by N. Becker,
1928. With her short,
Marcel-waved hair and her
slim, elegant figure, Mary
is dressed in a loose-fitting
ankle-length evening
dress.

Right
The Victorian skirt was
supported by a wire cage
– a crinoline – that took its
weight and replaced the
innumerable petticoats
and horsehair pads that
would have been worn to
create volume in the 1700s.
This particular example
also incorporates a bustle.

Mary might well have consigned Frances's clothing to the dressing up box!

Frances is also wearing more underwear than outerwear. It is easy to see that her upper body is rigidly corseted to allow her to achieve the shape required to fit into her dress. Her huge skirt is supported by a wire cage – a crinoline – which takes its weight and replaces the innumerable petticoats and horsehair pads that would have been worn to create volume by her predecessors in the previous century. As we can see in Mary's portrait, dresses became looser, narrower and simpler and, rather daringly, the corset was replaced by the brassiere. Mary looks far more relaxed and comfortable; she had already had three of her five children by the time this portrait was painted and would seem to be wearing little beneath her loosely belted dress other than a slip, drawers and the new-fangled brassiere.

The early eighteenth-century habit of wearing undergarments developed for reasons of personal cleanliness and also to avoid expensive clothes being soiled. Both men and women protected their expensive, heavily embroidered silk waistcoats, jackets or gowns from direct contact with bodily fluids by wearing cotton or linen next to the skin: a shirt for the likes of Topham Beauclerk and the 4th Duke; a shift for Lady Diana Russell and Lady Diana Beauclerk (both née Spencer).

Linen or cotton worked well for this purpose because laundering it was a straightforward matter: both fabrics could be boiled or bleached and this could be carried out in the Palace laundry. Expensive silks or woollens could not be washed without sustaining damage and so were sent to be dealt with by specialists. Silks were cleaned annually by

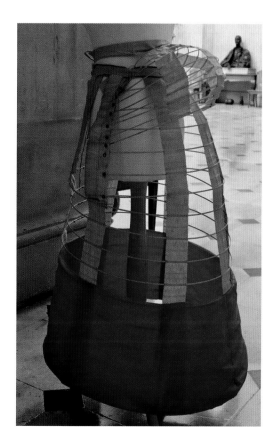

'scourers' who would spot clean garments using materials from their veritable arsenal of cleaning products, which included fuller's earth, chalk or salt to draw out oil and fat, lemon juice, vinegar and even urine.

Fuller's earth has been associated with the wool trade for thousands of years, both in the processing (the removal of excess lanolin) and later in the dry cleaning of woollen clothing. It is a natural claylike substance that has to be dug up from the ground. The final wool-making process to remove excess grease was known as 'fulling'. Those who carried out the work were known as 'fullers' and this name was later given to those involved in cleaning woollens. Dried teasels were the tools of a fuller's trade.

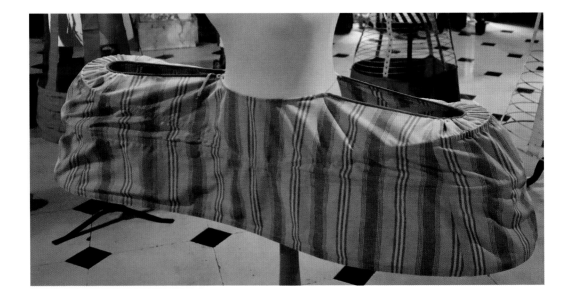

They would be used to loosen the fibres and this allowed the fuller's earth to fall easily from the garment, taking with it any dirt. A ledger entry for 1710 records the 1st Duke paying 10 shillings (50p) to have his 'cloaths' cleaned – over £80 today – which was quite a considerable amount for a single transaction.

Situated in the centre of the Palace on the south side is the Saloon, historically the formal dining room, where kings, queens and heads of state have been served course after course of delicious – and sometimes bizarre – food. It seemed perversely appropriate to display here the underclothing, whose constraints would have made eating a torture for some.

A lady's undergarments were somewhat complicated and numerous. As fashions changed, so too did the body shape required to display them to their best advantage, and therefore so did the underwear. Stays, hoops, corsets and crinolines were used to mould the body in such a way that the most impractical

and uncomfortable clothes could be worn.

It did not prove possible to display a genuine eighteenth-century hoop such as Duchess Sarah or her daughters and granddaughters wore, but help was at hand, this time from Ian Chipperfield 'The Stay-maker'. Using traditional methods and materials to produce period pieces, Ian is an expert in his field and made an extraordinary set of hoops for me. It was such fun to have the opportunity to try them on: one immediately begins to mince sideways, rather than walk normally. Ian was horrified and pointed out how ridiculous any self-respecting woman of fashion would look dressed in the finest silk gown, scuttling sideways like a crab. I quickly learned to glide at a jaunty angle and was soon able to pass through the enfilade doors without mishap.

Traditional hoops were made of linen and then horizontal hoops were sewn in at regular intervals to make them rigid, but collapsible. Their purpose was simply to hold out the skirt

Left

Traditional hoops were made of linen and then horizontal hoops were sewn in at regular intervals to make them rigid, but collapsible. Their purpose was simply to hold out the skirt of a robe at the sides and display its detail to the best advantage.

Right

The mantua was a formal, wide-hipped, open gown made from very fine wool or silk, typically embroidered with silver or gold thread. A matching train and petticoat would complete the look.

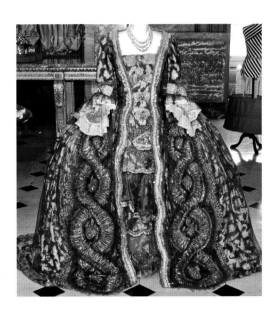

of a robe at the sides and display its detail to the best advantage. If one looked at a lady of fashion, she would appear to be a normal size sideways on, but extraordinarily wide (1.5 m or so) when viewed from the front.

Having a set of hoops was great, but having a mantua to demonstrate what the hoops would have supported made everything even better. The mantua was a formal, wide-hipped, open gown made from fine wool or silk, typically embroidered with silver or gold thread. A matching train and petticoat would have completed the look. Very few genuine examples of early eighteenth-century mantuas have survived. They were extremely impractical and eventually became unfashionable, except for court wear. The fabric for these dresses was so expensive that the majority were eventually unpicked and restyled according to the prevailing fashion of the day.

Given that this was the case, the generous contribution made by Philip Blake-Jones

of the London Festival Opera and Opera Intervals was especially welcome. I happened to be reading *the Sunday Times* Travel section one day (ever hopeful) when I glimpsed a photograph of two ladies in period costume. They were part of an opera company that entertained cruise passengers and they were wearing the most spectacular mantuas, one of which ended up in the Saloon at Blenheim Palace. The gown was simply magnificent and such a wonderful way to demonstrate exactly the job for which the hoops were designed.

If an eighteenth-century lady's mantua was supported by her hoops, then her stays were used to fashion the upper body into a rounded cone shape. They were more forgiving and comfortable to wear than the nineteenth-century corset, so much so that even children wore them, stiffened with cardboard rather than the more rigid metal or whalebone used in the construction of adult stays. Wealthy women wore their stays over a chemise and, as

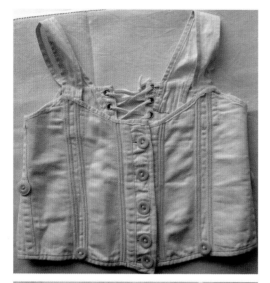

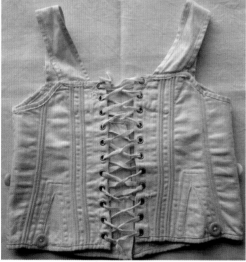

the outer layer was often made from decorative silk brocade, they would actually form part of the bodice of the gown.

Women from all ranks of society wore stays. Poorer women wore them for strength and support to help them carry out manual tasks. These stays would be made of fustian and laced at the front or sides so that they could fasten them themselves. A wealthy woman would wear stays 'for fashion', which were laced at the back; she had servants to make them secure. The very poorest women could not afford even the simplest of stays made from the plainest fabric, so their bodies remained loose rather than tightly bound, giving rise to the expression 'loose women': a reflection of a woman's economic status, not her morals.

A lady's stays would typically incorporate a busk, which was a loose length of flat wood, ivory or bone. It was inserted down the front of the stays to give extra support. As busks were worn next to the heart, they were often carved with initials and hearts or inset with tiny diamond-shaped mirrors and presented as love tokens by devoted husbands or lovers – or both!

Stay-making was an extremely skilful job, always carried out by a man. He would visit his clients to take detailed measurements and every part of the garment was hand sewn, even

The very poorest women could not afford even the simplest of stays made from the plainest fabric, so their bodies remained loose rather than tightly bound

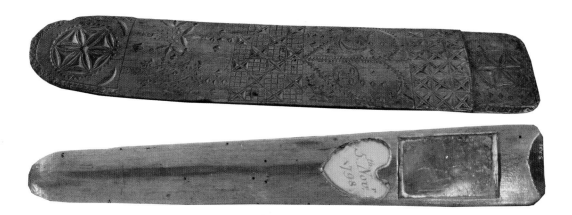

the tiny eyelets. The early sewing machine would eventually making an appearance in the mid-nineteenth century. Stays made from silks or brocades were expensive and therefore the prerogative of the rich; they would be mended rather than discarded or new ones made. Entries in the ledgers of the 4th Duke of Marlborough in 1790 show payments of 10 shillings (50p) for repairing and relining Lady Anne's stays, but only 3 shillings (15p) to adjust them. A new pair cost £2, which is considerably more than the butler's weekly wage of 86.5p, the equivalent of roughly £133 today.

During the nineteenth century, stays developed into corsets, as worn by Duchess Frances. The shape of the upper body changed from a rounded, tapering tube into

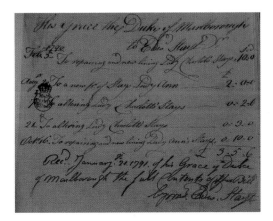

Left top
Even children wore stays. They would be stiffened with cardboard rather than the more rigid metal or whalebone used in the construction of adult stays.

Left below
These pink stays have been repaired with a darn – at the top left of the lacing – and have buttons to which leading reins could be attached.

Above Top
A lady's stays would typically incorporate a busk, which was a loose length of flat wood, ivory or bone. It was inserted down the front of the stays to give extra support.

Above middle
Busks were worn next to the heart so they were often carved with initials and hearts, or inset with tiny diamond-shaped mirrors and presented as love tokens by devoted husbands or lovers.

Above below
Stays were expensive to make and mend. Entries in the ledgers of the 4th Duke of Marlborough in 1790 show payments of 10 shillings (50p) for repairing and relining Lady Anne's stays, but only 3 shillings (15p) to adjust them. A new pair cost £2, which is considerably more than the butler's weekly wage of 86.5p.

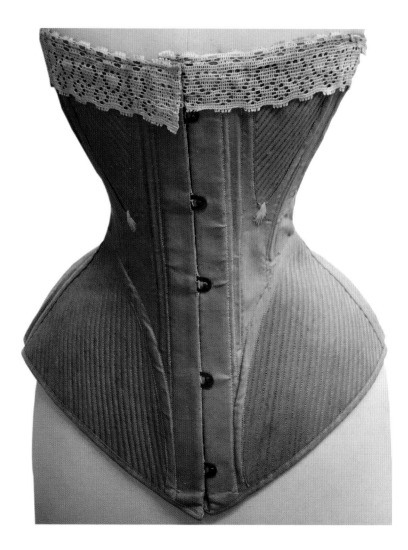

Left
During the nineteenth century, stays developed into corsets. The shape of the upper body changed from a rounded, tapering tube into a far more curved and rigid form, which produced a tiny waist and accentuated the bosom. Corsets like this could give the wearer a 49.5-cm waist.

a far more curved and rigid form, which produced a tiny waist and accentuated the bosom. The earlier type of stay busk was replaced with a two-part corset busk made from metal. One half of the busk would have a hook and the other an eye so that it was easier for the wearer to put on or remove.

In the mid-1800s skirts that had narrowed and become far simpler during the earlier part of the century became increasingly wide. At first they were supported by layers of petticoats and bustles, the petticoats being made from a cotton and horsehair fabric called 'crin' (French for horsehair). This arrangement was both heavy and unhygienic and it was eventually replaced by the crinoline. Typically a cage constructed from wire hoops, there were also versions that had tubes made from caoutchouc rubber, which could then be inflated to the required dimensions.

The crinoline remained popular until the 1870s when the crinolette found favour. This was a flat-fronted version of the crinoline with additional support at the rear. Eventually, bustle pads were also used to give extra volume at the rear. These were filled with straw or horsehair and made it difficult for the wearer to sit comfortably. All was not lost, however. Enter the 'Keelapso' bustle: specially designed and resembling a mini-crinoline, it would gracefully collapse as the lady took her seat. What bliss!

Gentlemen's undergarments have always been far less complicated than a lady's and therefore a simple matter to portray. Until the twentieth century, a shirt was considered to be underwear and it was very bad manners for a gentleman to display anything of it in public, other than the collar, cuffs and a little of the front. Breeches served a double purpose as both underwear and outerwear, and boasted a buttoned flap at the front that made life easier. I had obtained an eighteenth-century linen shirt, but alas no period breeches. An earlier exhibition, *Lights, Camera, Action!* had necessitated a trip to a well-known London costumier and, while looking for costumes used at Blenheim for the filming of Kenneth Branagh's *Hamlet*, I came across a pair of breeches that had been worn by Colin Firth in the BBC's definitive production of *Pride and Prejudice*. I had not been able to justify hiring them at the time as, although Blenheim Palace is mentioned once in the book, there is no real connection. This time, however, I felt fully justified in securing the only item in the entire exhibition for which we had to pay. It was worth it for the sheer joy of seeing Mr Darcy's breeches every day for four months!

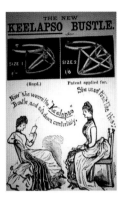

Right
Advertisement for *'The New Keelapso Bustle'*, *The Illustrated London News*, 18 June 1887. Bustle pads were used to give extra volume at the rear. These were filled with straw or horsehair and made it difficult for the wearer to sit comfortably. Enter the 'Keelapso' bustle, specially designed for comfort: resembling a mini-crinoline, it would gracefully collapse as the lady took her seat.

Below
Until the twentieth century, a shirt was considered to be underwear and it was very bad manners for a gentleman to display anything of it in public, other than the collar, cuffs and a little of the front. Breeches served a double purpose as both underwear and outerwear, and boasted a buttoned flap at the front that made life easier.

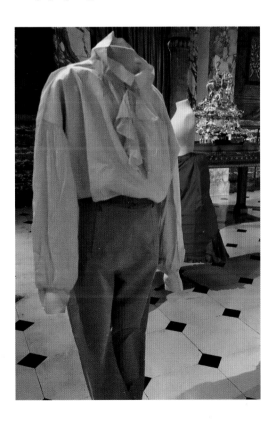

CHAPTER 8

Fashion to die for

A sinister danger lurked in every fashionable Paris Green gown

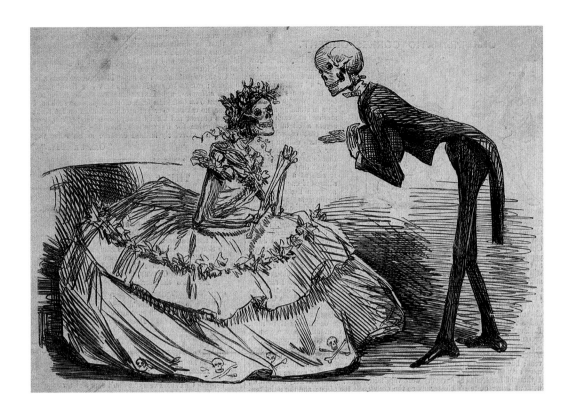

True fashionistas have always been prepared to go to extremes in order to stay at the cutting edge of fashion. The wig-wearers of the eighteenth century exposed themselves to all sorts of dangers, not least from the suppliers of the expensive powder used to complete the must-have hairstyle of the moment. Some suppliers went to extremes to hoodwink their clients and a report in *The Times* dated 29 July 1786 tells the woeful story of a gentleman playing cards. He leaned his wig too close to the candle, not realising that the powder that had been applied to his stylish wig had been mixed with gunpowder. As well as injuring his fellow card players, the resulting explosion burnt the gentleman's head so badly that, 'the skin of the head and back part of the neck peeled off entirely and the sutures of the skull were as plainly to be discovered as in a skeleton. It is said he is [unsurprisingly] since dead.'

Duchess Frances followed the fashion of the times. She trimmed her waist down to tiny proportions by wearing a tightly laced corset, which she could let out to accommodate her 11 pregnancies. Frances and women like her would have found that corset-wearing displaced their inner organs and could refashion their ribs and spine: all so that they might achieve their goal of a 38-cm waist. The Victorian lady would risk feeling continually faint and breathless. It is perhaps no wonder that so many of them were prone to regular fits of the vapours and that members of the medical

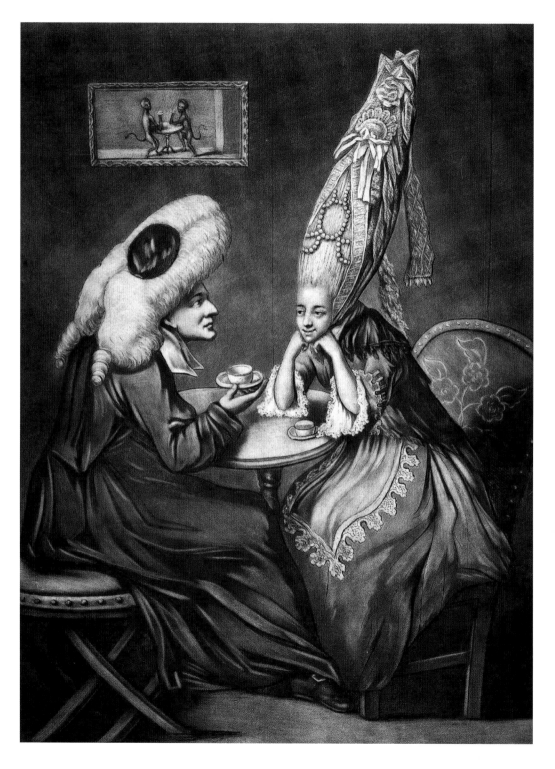

profession published dire warnings of the onset of ailments such as cancer, consumption, hysteria and epilepsy as a consequence of wearing corsets and of lacing them too tightly.

Neither was the wearing of the crinoline without danger or inconvenience. There are endless nineteenth-century newspaper reports of women falling over and being unable to get up, and of indignant male churchgoers who would find themselves sharing a pew with crinoline-wearing ladies and being enveloped in their skirts. Gentlemen sometimes had to ride on the outside of their own carriages in the pouring rain in order to oblige ladies 'hedged in their shells like the clapper of a bell'. There is even a report in *The Times* regarding the wedding of the Princess Royal on 1 January 1858, when the private entrance to the Chapel Royal at St James's Palace was widened by 60 cm to allow Queen Victoria and her daughter access, the work being carried out so that the entrance was 'capable of admitting crinoline of any amplitude!'.

Very occasionally, a crinoline would prove to be a lifesaver: take, for example, the case of the unfortunate Martha Sheppard, a seventeen-year-old who thought she would end it all by leaping off the bridge over the Serpentine in Hyde Park. She had reckoned without the ballooning effect of her crinoline, which acted as a buoyancy aid and kept her afloat just long enough for her to be rescued by a passing constable.

Others were not so fortunate. People tripped over crinolines in the street and fell into the path of horse-drawn vehicles; women were crushed by factory machinery; and a woman on Clapham Common was struck by lightning and killed, her metal busk and wire crinoline acting

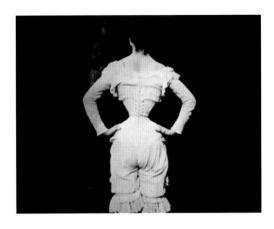

Previous page
The Arsenic Waltz, Punch, 8 February 1862.

Left
Miss Prattle Consulting Doctor Double Fee about her Pantheon Head Dress, published by Carington Bowles, c. 1771. It is easy to see how a powdered wig if coming into contact with a naked flame might bear explosive

results, particularly if the powder had been mixed with gunpowder by an unscrupulous merchant.

Above
Corset-wearing displaced a woman's inner organs and could refashion her ribs and spine: all so that she might achieve her goal of a 38-cm waist, as seen here in a photograph from c. 1890.

At the 1858 wedding of the Princess Royal, the private entrance to the Chapel Royal at St James's Palace had to be widened to allow the crinoline-wearing Queen Victoria to enter

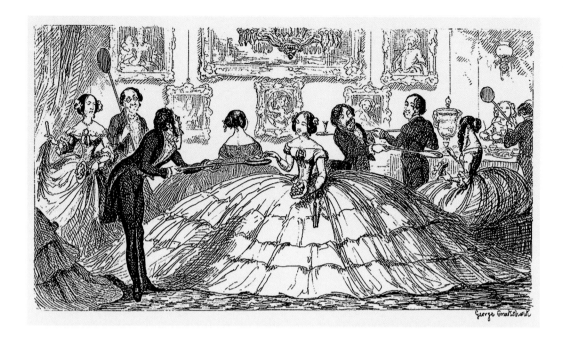

as excellent conductors. More common are the numerous reports and graphic descriptions of women's voluminous skirts being set alight when coming into contact with open fires or burning candles and of the poor souls dying in agony. The cages beneath the skirts fanned the flames as effectively as any set of bellows and the fires took hold in minutes.

A letter to *The Times* dated 6 December 1858, from a reader whose wife had narrowly escaped death in this manner, implores the newspaper to campaign against 'this dangerous tyranny of fashion' so that he might enjoy without fear the 'blazing hearths' that would warm the winter ahead.

By the end of the nineteenth century the crinoline was no longer fashionable, although there was a move to resurrect it. A 'No Crinoline League' was formed with an initial 5,625 members and readers of *The Times* took to

their pens to encourage English women who valued their lives to 'keep the accursed thing at a distance'. Fortunately, they heeded the advice.

A more sinister danger lurked in the very fabric of ladies' gowns and adornments. During the nineteenth century emerald, or Paris green, became the colour of choice for the fashion conscious. Unfortunately, the colour was created by using a dye containing arsenite of copper and anything containing even a hint of arsenic was always going to be a problem.

The dye from the tinted fabrics was easily absorbed into the skin when the wearer perspired or, if it had not been fixed correctly, when traces of powder fell directly onto the skin. This type of arsenic poisoning gave rise to rashes, sores, vomiting and nausea, but fortunately the ill effects did not last once the dress had been removed. The men and women involved in the manufacturing

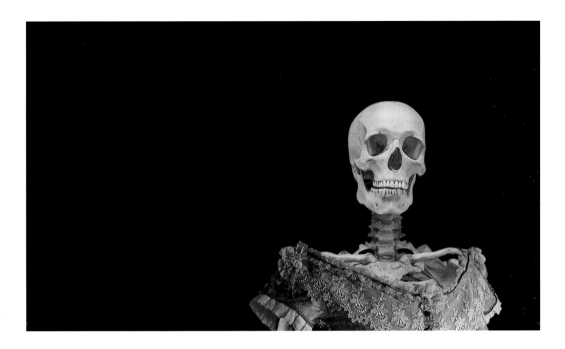

left

A Splendid Spread, by George Cruikshank, from *The Comic Almanack,* 1850. The crinoline reached ridiculous – and dangerous – proportions. There are numerous reports and graphic descriptions of women's voluminous skirts setting alight when coming into contact with open fires or burning candles. The cages beneath the skirts fanned the flames as effectively as any set of bellows and fire took hold in minutes.

Above

During the nineteenth century emerald, or Paris green, became the popular colour of choice. Unfortunately, the colour was created by using a dye containing arsenite of copper and anything containing even a hint of arsenic was always going to be a problem.

process were not so lucky. Following the death in 1861 of Matilda Scheurer, a nineteen-year-old artificial-flower maker, the Ladies' Sanitary Association called for an inquiry to be made into her death and into the whole manufacturing and dyeing process. The results did not make for comfortable reading. The men who actually manufactured the powder often worked in the open air and would merely suffer from boils, pimples, itching and sneezing. These symptoms would subside once they were at a distance from their workplace and so no great importance was attached to them.

There were known risks associated with the manufacture of green cloth, but far greater was the danger involved in the production of artificial flowers, which were widely in demand to trim hats, gowns and headdresses. This was because the dye in powder form had to be handled so frequently in the creation of leaves and foliage. The shapes were cut from muslin and the dye was dusted onto them using a small muslin bag. Some of the leaves were then dipped in wax, which would fix the dye and make it relatively safe; those where the dye was not fixed were known as 'fluffed' leaves and were literally poisonous.

The women used what methods they could to avoid coming into direct contact with the powder. They would cover their mouths and nostrils with a towel, or raise their aprons and tie them around the lower half of their faces, but these were nominal precautions. The effects of coming into regular contact with the powdered pigment were severe. What would seem to start off as a cold quickly turned into something far more sinister: stomach cramps, vomiting, diarrhoea, nose bleeds, pustules, open sores, hair loss and raging ulcers, particularly on the fingers.

A report into the use of arsenic was published in 1862 by a Dr Guy for the Medical Office of the Privy Council and in it he made several recommendations. Generally, he believed that the effects were 'disagreeable, even painful' but because they 'subsided...without leaving... permanent disability' he did not ban the use of arsenic-based dyes, other than in food colouring (sweets, apple tarts, blancmanges). Green wall hangings and wrapping paper had to be stamped with the words 'arsenical paper', and the only other restriction was that factory owners were not allowed to use workers aged eighteen or under, particularly for 'fluffing'. The general tone was that since there had only been one actual death directly linked to arsenic poisoning, then a little inconvenience to the employees was something that had to be borne.* Perhaps this accounts for the colour

green being thought unlucky even today.

Arsenic was not the only harmful substance in use in the fashion industry. Felt was employed extensively in hat-making: not the type of felt we think of today, which is often green and bought by the metre, but felt produced from animal pelts. Animals such as beavers met the demand for the beaver hats much loved by nineteenth-century gentlemen; rabbit pelts were used for the cheaper versions worn by the lower orders.

In order to produce felt, the fur had to be separated from the skin, but care had to be taken to keep it intact, so that it could then be moulded easily into shape. An orange-coloured mixture was used to do this in a process that, rather appropriately, was known as 'carroting'. Unfortunately, the mixture contained mercury and, as it was heated, it would give off a strong vapour. The ill effects of working with mercury in this way were not recognised until the end of the nineteenth century; for some time, mercury was even prescribed for medical purposes to cure diseases such as syphilis.

It was eventually realised that prolonged exposure to the vapour, particularly in confined spaces, gave rise to numerous complaints, including hair loss, bleeding gums, drooling, tremors and madness, which, undoubtedly, is how Lewis Carroll ended up with a Mad Hatter in his classic novel of 1865.

---

*From the article 'The Use of Arsenic as a Colour', The Times, 4 September 1863.

Below
John Tenniel's drawing of the
Mad Hatter reciting his nonsense
poem 'Twinkle Twinkle Little
Bat', from Lewis Carroll's *Alice's
Adventures in Wonderland*. Felt
is employed extensively for
hat-making. The use of mercury
in the felting process gave rise to
numerous complaints, including
hair loss, bleeding gums, drooling,
tremors and madness, which,
undoubtedly, is how Carroll ended
up with a Mad Hatter in his classic
novel of 1865.

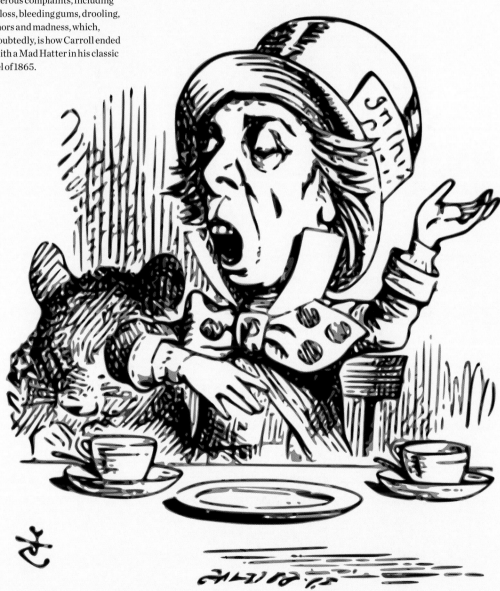

CHAPTER 9

The Victorian Royal House Party

'The number of changes of costume in itself was a waste of time…one was not supposed to wear the same gown twice'

Consuelo, the 9th Duchess, referring to a typical day when hosting a Royal house party

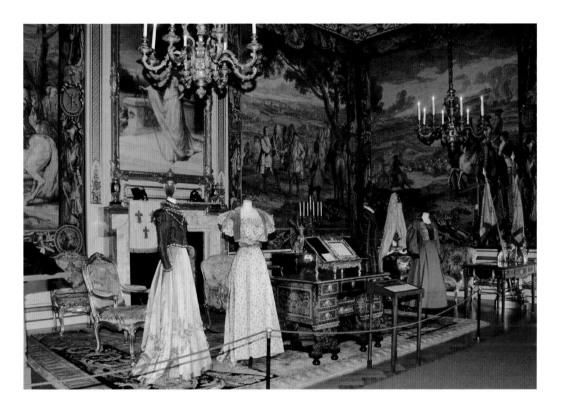

Consuelo Vanderbilt was born into one of America's wealthiest families in March 1877 and hers was undoubtedly a life of great privilege. As a sixteen-year-old, she travelled to Europe with her overbearing mother, Alva, and it was in Paris that she enjoyed her first ball. In preparation for this important event, mother and daughter had visited the leading couturiers of the city and this resulted in Consuelo arriving at the ball in a tightly laced and corseted white tulle gown created for her by the House of Worth. It was at this Parisian ball that she met her future husband, Jacques Balsan, although that particular wedding would not take place for almost thirty years.

From Paris the Vanderbilts travelled on to London and, before they returned to New York in the autumn of 1894, they met with a number of fellow Americans, among them Lady Randolph Churchill (Jennie Jerome) and the godmother after whom Consuelo was named, Consuelo Yznaga, Duchess of Manchester and one of the earliest 'Dollar Princesses'. It was at this time that Consuelo Vanderbilt also met Charles Spencer-Churchill, the 9th Duke of Marlborough, another of her future husbands. This marriage, however, would take place in just over a year.

Alva and Consuelo returned to London in 1895, shortly after Consuelo's 18th birthday. After renewing their acquaintance with the 9th Duke at a ball, he quickly despatched an invitation for them to visit Blenheim Palace.

Consuelo's initial impressions of Blenheim were akin to those of Elizabeth Bennet on viewing Pemberley for the first time: who could help but be struck by its magnificence? However, there the similarity ends. Whereas Elizabeth had by this point warmed considerably towards Mr Darcy, Consuelo departed Blenheim with the firm opinion that marriage to the duke was out of the question, particularly as by now she considered herself to be secretly engaged to a fellow American.

She had reckoned without the machinations of her ambitious mother!

An invitation was duly sent to the duke asking him to visit the Vanderbilts at their Newport home. It was readily accepted so Consuelo gathered her courage to tell her mother of her love for Winthrop Rutherfurd, a fellow New Yorker and sportsman, whom she had met before they departed on their tour of Europe. Alva took to her bed with a fit

of the vapours, palpitations and every other weapon in her armoury and Consuelo, being of a biddable nature, felt that the only course of action open to her was to renounce her first love and eventually accept the proposal of the Duke of Marlborough when it was later made during his September visit.

To say that Consuelo was a reluctant bride is something of an understatement. She married the 9th Duke of Marlborough on 6 November 1895. The marriage of this beautiful eighteen-year-old heiress to one of the country's most eligible bachelors received almost as much press coverage then, both in the UK and the US, as did the marriage of Prince Harry to Meghan Markle in May 2018.

Numerous paragraphs in the press were devoted to descriptions of the bridal party, particularly of Consuelo's dress, which Alva

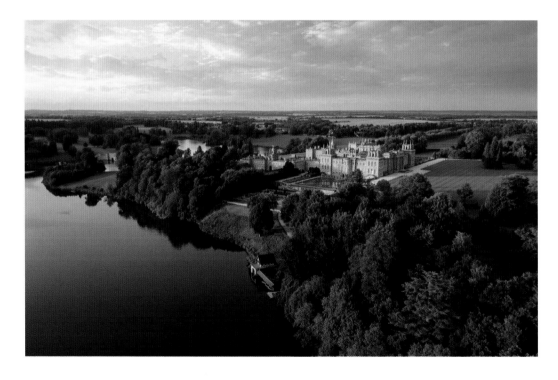

had had the foresight to order on their earlier visit to Paris, so certain was she that her plan for Consuelo to marry into the British aristocracy would be a success.

The newspaper reports were mixed. The bride looked stunning in her white satin dress with its tiers of Brussels lace, high collar and wide sleeves narrowing below the elbow. Her train was the regulation 4.5 m long and fell from her shoulders. Its border was trimmed with pearls and tiny silver rose leaves interspaced – ironically – with lovers' knots. It lent itself perfectly to being refashioned the following year to be worn when Consuelo was presented at court.

Many newspaper reports contained a great deal of censure, however, especially as it was felt that this was a marriage of convenience and even more American dollars would be lost from the local economy. One newspaper reported wryly that the duke had bought a pair of cotton socks on his visit, so at least some of Consuelo's millions would be remaining on American soil.

The happy couple were unable to return to Blenheim immediately after the wedding as a great deal of restoration was taking place at the Palace, paid for with Consuelo's dowry. The duke was not greatly travelled at this point in his life, so the newlyweds set off for the Mediterranean and took in areas of Italy and Spain before eventually making their way to Paris. Consuelo availed herself of the opportunity to revisit the House of Worth, where she was welcomed and her many purchases overseen by Jean-Philippe Worth himself.

The 9th Duke and Consuelo finally reached Blenheim Palace in March 1896, shortly after Consuelo's nineteenth birthday. They were

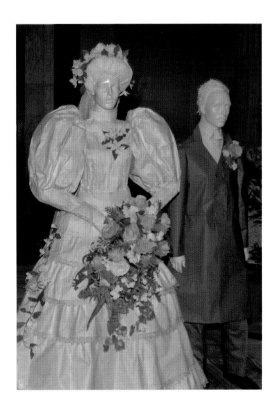

Previous page
The First State Room was used as an anteroom by visiting royal guests. It provided the perfect backdrop for a range of frocks that would typically be worn over the space of just one day.

Left
Consuelo's initial impressions of Blenheim Palace were akin to those of Elizabeth Bennet on viewing Pemberley for the first time: who could help but be struck by its magnificence?

Above
The bride looked stunning in her white satin dress with its tiers of Brussels lace, high collar and wide sleeves narrowing below the elbow. Her train was the regulation 4.5 m long and fell from her shoulders. Here it is reproduced faithfully in paper by Denise Watson.

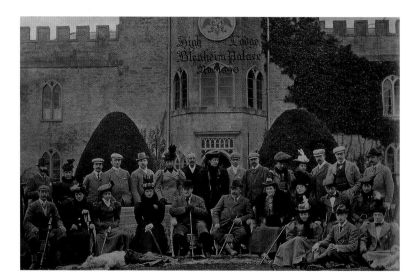

Left
A weekend shooting party
in November 1896. The
9th Duke and Consuelo's
guests included the Prince
of Wales – later King
Edward VII (sixth from the
left on the the front row) –
and Winston Churchill's
mother, Jennie Jerome
(seated second from the
left on the same row).

greeted with great enthusiasm by tenants and townsfolk alike, all anxious to catch their first glimpse of the new American duchess.

Life at Blenheim Palace held many challenges for the young Consuelo, not least playing hostess to weekend house-party guests, which over a weekend in November 1896 included notables such as the Prince of Wales (later King Edward VII) and Winston Churchill's mother, Jennie Jerome. The sober-faced members of the royal party and other guests were photographed sitting outside High Lodge, a building towards the north of the Park, designed by Capability Brown, where once stood the home in which the dissolute Earl of Rochester (played by Johnny Depp in *The Libertine*) was found dead.

One of the many concerns faced by Consuelo was the protocol involved in such royal visits. She would ponder at length about appropriate seating arrangements – who should be seated next to whom – and also consider how she could overcome the problem of providing hot baths

for all her guests in a Palace greatly lacking in bathrooms. On occasions such as these, the Blenheim maids would not only be expected to house visiting staff in their quarters, but also to help provide water for over thirty baths a day. It is no wonder that one of the first things Consuelo's daughter-in-law did when her husband became 10th Duke was to convert some of the redundant powder rooms into bathrooms.

A further strain was knowing what to wear each day. These weekend visits would generally be of a four-day duration and Consuelo and her female guests, the leaders of fashion at the time, were expected to have four changes of outfit for each day.

The First State Room – part of a suite of three rooms – was used as an anteroom for only the most important of guests. Today the room is dominated by Carolus-Duran's portrait of a young, innocent-looking Consuelo dressed in a white dress, just as she had been for her first ball in Paris, only a few years previously.

Right
The First State Room is
dominated by Carolus-
Duran's portrait of c.
1893 of a young, innocent-
looking Consuelo dressed
in a white dress, just as she
had been for her first ball
in Paris, only a few years
before coming to Blenheim
as a bride.

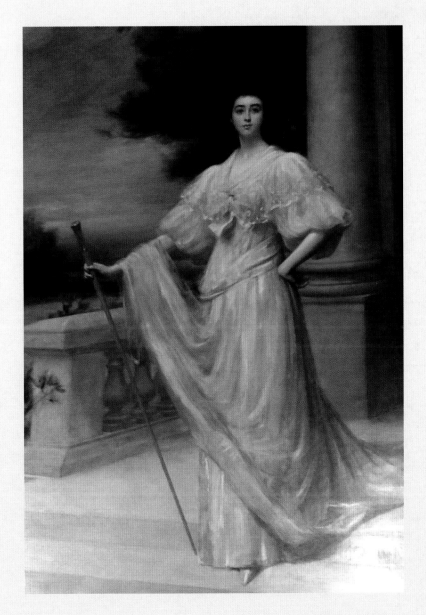

This seemed the ideal setting to display a typical array of dresses that the Victorian lady would have worn on just one day during the Prince of Wales's visit. Each lady would have had to pack at least sixteen different outfits for the duration of the four-day visit, plus the appropriate accessories, jewellery, petticoats and corsets. One further essential the lady guest would need for her Blenheim visit was a personal maid. How else could she possibly manipulate the button hooks, boot hooks and glove stretchers needed to fasten buttons, pull on boots or tease the fingers of kid gloves apart so that they would be just wide enough for a delicate hand to be slipped carefully inside?

In her memoir, *The Glitter and the Gold* (1952), Consuelo wrote:

> breakfast demanded an elegant costume of velvet or silk...we next changed into tweeds to join the [men]...an elaborate tea gown was donned for tea, after which we played cards or listened to...the organ until time to dress for dinner, when we adorned ourselves in satin or brocade... Clearly a tedious business!

Sadly, although Consuelo did her duty and provided the 9th Duke with two sons – an heir and a spare – the marriage was not to last and ended in divorce. It was not until 1921 that Consuelo eventually married Jacques Balsan, the young man who had been smitten by her at that first Parisian ball and who had confidently informed his mother, even then, that he had met the girl he was going to marry. Theirs was a long and happy marriage and, although they had no children together, the couple played a huge part in the lives of Consuelo's children and grandchildren for the many years they spent together.

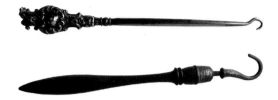

Above top
A button hook: an essential accessory for any Victorian woman and her maid.

Above bottom
A boot hook: vital for pulling on tightly fitting boots.

Below
Consuelo: 'breakfast demanded an elegant costume of velvet or silk... we next changed into tweeds to join the [men]...'.

Right
'an elaborate tea gown was donned for tea, after which we played cards or listened to...the organ until time to dress for dinner, when we adorned ourselves in satin or brocade...'. The fitted jacket and dress would have been worn for tea in the afternoon, while the slightly more revealing short-sleeved dress with the lower neckline would be donned for the evening.

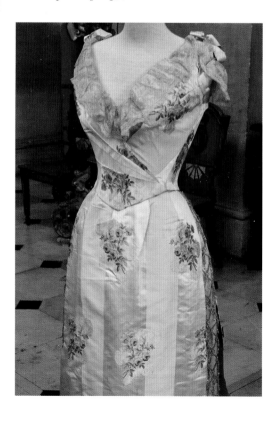

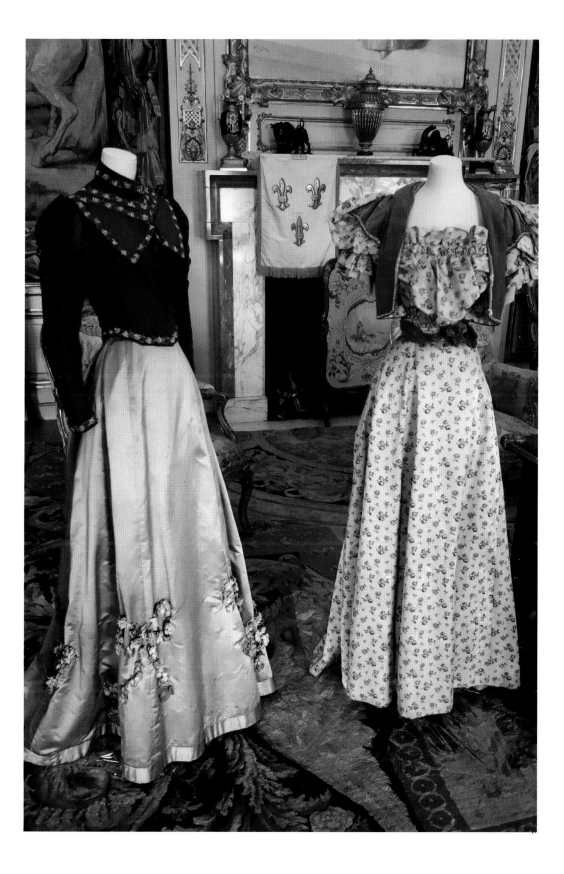

CHAPTER 10

Shoes: An Evolution

'The real proof of an elegant woman is what is on her feet'

Christian Dior

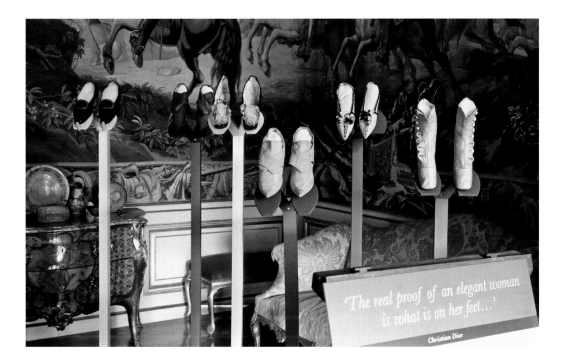

'The real proof of an elegant woman is what is on her feet...'

Christian Dior

W e have been wearing things on our feet to protect them and keep them warm since time immemorial. Over time, footwear was adapted so that it became not only functional, but also a way of demonstrating one's wealth, status and aspirations. As this occurred, functionality sometimes went out of the window – as it does today – and both men and women would suffer great discomfort to follow the latest fashion in footwear.

The lavish Second State Room at Blenheim Palace is one of the best rooms in the house and was once used as a sitting room for royal and other high-ranking visitors. It is dominated, rather unusually, by a huge painting of Louis XIV, who was king of France at the time of the 1st Duke of Marlborough's defeat of the French at the Battle of Blenheim in 1704.

The painting portrays Louis seated (he was very conscious of his lack of height) wearing clothes made from the most luxurious and expensive fabrics, and an exquisite pair of be-ribboned shoes. Louis XIV was rather vain and extremely proud of his manly calves, which he shows off to great effect. He frequently sported shoes with red heels that served to draw attention to his beautifully shaped feet and also as a symbol of his belief that his court at Versailles was higher than 'the rest of humanity'.

Legend has it that the idea of wearing red heels came to Louis XIV after visiting an abattoir where the blood from the floor soaked into the heels on the shoes he was wearing. Instead of flying into a rage, he was rather pleased with the overall effect and had the red heel developed as a fashion statement. Ever mindful of wishing to stand apart from the lower orders, he passed a sumptuary law

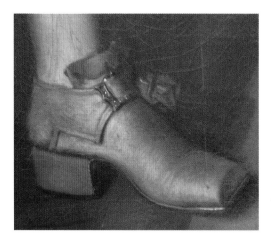

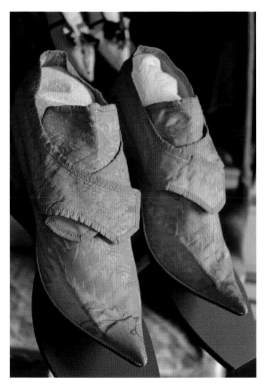

forbidding anyone other than members of the aristocracy from wearing red-heeled shoes. He even had a particular type of waisted high heel, 'the Louis', named after him.

The red heel eventually became one of the most popular and widespread trends in Europe and was seen in the English court just as frequently as it had been in France. Ironically, the trend became a favourite even among the family and friends of Louis XIV's sworn enemy, the 1st Duke of Marlborough. A number of his grandsons and great-grandson elected to wear them in their portraits, so that they could be admired for posterity.

What better place to display the wonderful range of shoes, spanning two centuries, than under the appreciative nose of Louis XIV!

Two pairs of women's shoes – one in yellow figured satin and the other in ribbed green silk –were among the oldest on display and dated from the mid-1700s. The delicate fabric from which they are made would have been protected by overshoes or by being elevated from the dirty streets by the use of pattens, which would raise the wearer (and her skirts) so that she and her shoes were not contaminated by the filth that

ran freely in public places. Pattens were mostly worn by women, and for wealthier ladies they were made to match their shoes, thus enabling patten-makers to develop their skills in embroidery and other decorative crafts.

Patten-makers, like many other craftsmen, were represented by a trade association called the Worshipful Guild of Pattenmakers. Their talents were being used mainly for the benefit of women and therefore the guild's motto was rather appropriately Recipiunt Fœminæ Sustentacula Nobis, which translates from the Latin as 'Women receive support from us', as indeed they did, right up until the mid-1800s when street paving and plumbing improved and the public was no longer faced with the chore of wading through the horse excrement (or worse) that filled the streets.

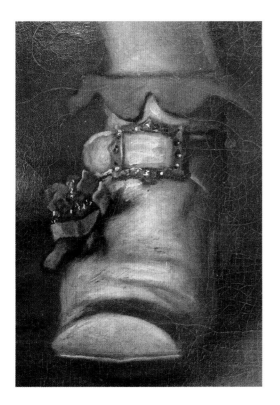

Both of these early pairs of shoes are similar in style, having delicate leather soles, 'waisted' heels and straight latchets, which would have been fastened with a buckle. They would have been made to match or complement a particular outfit and created at a time when shoes were not fashioned specifically for the left or right foot: as the shoe was worn it would eventually begin to mould to one foot or the other. This was the case particularly when shoes were made from materials such as soft, kid leather, silk or satin and the fashion was for 'straight' shoes.

Shoes were helpfully marked 'L' or 'R' – or 'droite' and 'gauche' in the case of models bought from France – as a reminder of which shoe went on which foot. This practice of not making shoes specifically for one foot or the other remained in force until the mid-1800s,

when contemporary styles dictated the need for shoemakers to use one last for the left foot and one for the right. Regular customers had the advantage of finding that the shoemaker would keep a last as a pattern for their feet and such was his skill, aptitude and intimate knowledge of a client's foot that he would be capable of patching footwear to accommodate the corns and bunions that wearing fashionable (or ill-fitting) shoes often caused.

Other period shoes on display included an exquisite pair of fine, soft, leather shoes in yellow and black with ribbon decoration. Dating back to the late 1700s, these beautiful and contemporary looking shoes benefited from a low 'peg' or 'Italian' heel. Shoes such as these would have been ordered to match a specific gown and worn with stockings that gave

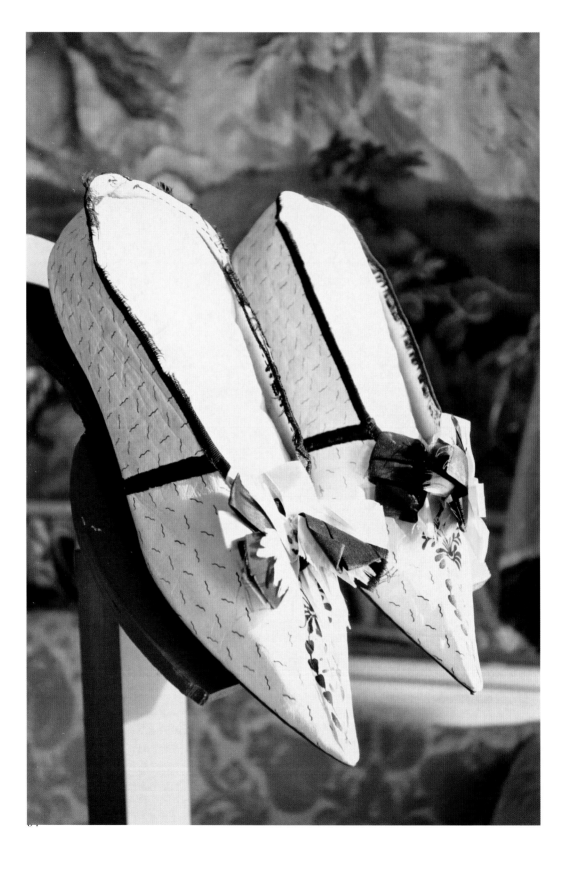

a glimpse of exquisite, tantalising embroidery at the ankle, coloured to match the leather from which they were made: the very thing for Caroline, 4th Duchess of Marlborough, and her lovely daughters.

The early years of the nineteenth century brought a further change in style in the form of plain, flat, half-boots (the Adelaide) or flat slippers, which remained hidden beneath the longer hemlines and became de rigueur for women, often in white leather for daywear and black for evening. Leather, originally associated with the lower orders, was now much appreciated by fashionable society, which came to appreciate the value of greater comfort and protection for the foot.

Some nineteenth-century flat boots could be worn today and easily pass for the Chelsea boot that continues to enjoy great popularity. This style was developed by Queen Victoria's bootmaker, Joseph Sparkes Hall, who in 1837 designed a flat half-boot with an elasticated side gusset (also known as the Garibaldi), which gave the lady the advantage of being able to slip it on and off relatively quickly and easily without the need for additional help from maid or boot hook.

Flat boots or slippers remained fashionable until the mid-1800s when heels began to creep up in height again. Winston Churchill's grandmother, Duchess Frances – she of the heavily corseted body – would have had the choice of a wide variety of styles ranging from rosette-decorated shoes to buttoned half-boots. These half-boots were fiddly to fasten with their tight laces or tiny buttons and made on very narrow lasts so that a lady's foot would always appear to be dainty and shapely. Women's feet became almost as uncomfortable as their

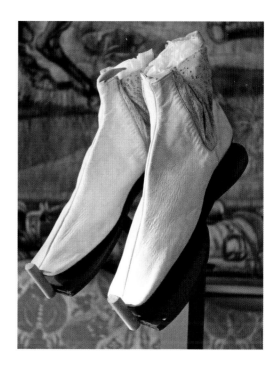

Left
An exquisite pair of fine, soft, leather shoes in yellow and black with ribbon decoration. These beautiful, contemporary looking kid leather shoes date back to the late 1700s.

Above
This popular style was developed by Queen Victoria's bootmaker, Joseph Sparkes Hall, who in 1837 designed a flat half-boot with an elasticated side gusset (also known as the Garibaldi).

corseted bodies. These latest styles put paid to the relative ease and comfort that women had enjoyed while wearing their Garibaldi boots.

The beginning of the twentieth century saw many changes. Queen Victoria's sixty-three-and-a-half-year reign finally came to an end and paved the way for the new, but brief, Edwardian era. The Prince of Wales, who had visited Blenheim as a guest of the 9th Duke and his new American wife, now became Edward VII, although his reign was to last a fraction of that of his mother. Edward was succeeded by his son George V in 1910 and it was during this Georgian era that Europe experienced the long, dark and devastating years of the First World War.

Women's fashions had not really varied drastically in style for hundreds of years. That altered with the advent of the First World War, when there were radical changes in a relatively short time. During the war, women were employed in traditional male roles in munitions factories or making aircraft parts; they had no use for the cumbersome crinolines, suffocating corsets or complicated coiffeurs of the Victorian and Edwardian eras. Short hair, considered ugly prior to the war, was regarded as a necessity for the safety of certain factory workers and this practical hairstyle was adapted by ladies of fashion as we saw earlier in the elegant portrait of the 10th Duchess.

The most lasting change at this time, however, was seen in women's hemlines, which rose from floor length to ankle length prior to the war and then to mid-calf by 1916. Hemlines have remained at that length and shorter ever since. This rather saucy change had a significant impact on shoe styles. As hemlines crept upwards, shoes became prettier and increasingly more decorative and colourful, especially for evening wear.

In the world of fashion, the past is never dead: some features merely rest in between repeat appearances. Louis XIV was famed for his decorative shoes with their red heels, but today the colour red when associated with shoes brings only one name to mind: Christian Louboutin.

The French designer's elegant and glamorous creations with their red, lacquered soles are among the most sought-after, aspirational and instantly recognisable brands in the world today. What shoe could be more appropriate to sit in solemn state beneath the portrait of the

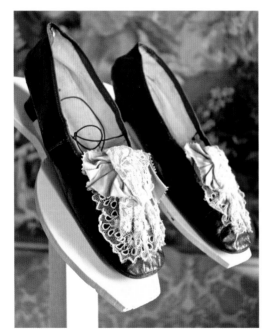

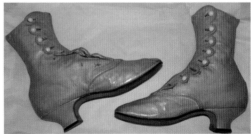

Left
By the mid-1800s, ladies had the choice of a wide variety of styles ranging from rosette-decorated shoes to buttoned half-boots.

Above
These half-boots would have been very fiddly to fasten with their tiny buttons. They were made on narrow lasts so that the lady's feet would always appear dainty and shapely.

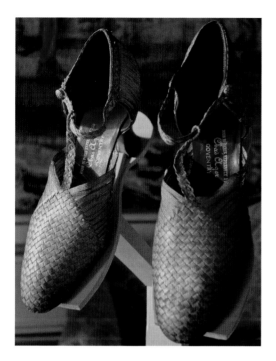

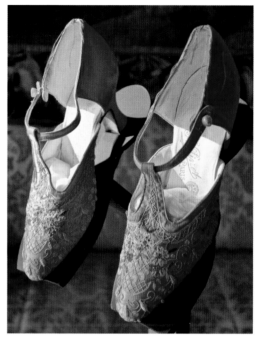

Sun King at Blenheim Palace?

I had had a great amount of luck in sourcing loans from many diverse quarters. I had the kind offer of various pairs of Louboutins from family, friends, even friends of friends, but the slight drawback was that each pair had been worn and, over time, the distinctive red soles had become scuffed. After a number of attempts, I managed to contact the correct

Above
As hemlines crept upwards after the end of the First World War, shoes became prettier and increasingly more decorative and colourful, especially for evening wear.

Above right
The most lasting change at the beginning of the

twentieth century was seen in women's hemlines, which rose from floor length to ankle length prior to the First World War and then to mid-calf by 1916. Hemlines have remained at that length and shorter ever since and had a significant impact on shoe styles.

person within the PR department at Christian Louboutin. She agreed to let me have a pair of shoes from the Louboutin archive and from then on the Louboutin team was so generous that nothing seemed too much trouble.

My eventual contact generously asked me which particular style of shoe I would like to borrow. Each shoe or boot is a work of art in itself and Louboutin has many followers who collect them as others collect paintings. In all honesty I had little idea about the styles available and so I jumped at the chance when she offered to send me the Louboutin 'catalogue' (I use the term lightly) so that I could make my choice.

I joined Blenheim in 2008 and since then I have moved desk at least six times: believe it or not, we are incredibly short of office space at the Palace. While undertaking research for

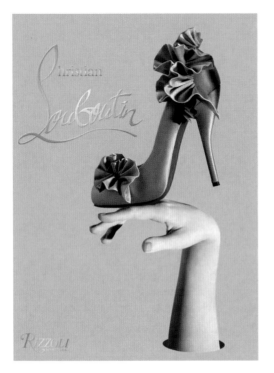

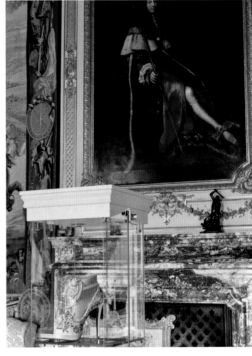

A Passion for Fashion, I worked at a desk in the Group Sales office with two very good friends, Cathy (Ted) Penry and Linda (Bijou) Fisher. I asked them to look out for post addressed to me – an A5 or even A4 envelope perhaps – but nothing arrived. After a further day or two, I had a call from our Estate office in nearby Woodstock: a package had arrived addressed to me and it was enormous! It contained the superb autobiography of Christian Louboutin and a pictorial record of the most incredible collection of shoes and boots I have ever seen. This huge leather-bound tome was amazing. Catalogue indeed!

Cathy, Linda and I spent a happy hour or so weighing up the merits of various styles: we each had our favourites, but how to decide on just one style? And then I saw it. The Marie-Antoinette. A masterpiece with a fastener

Above left
The superb autobiography of Christian Louboutin contains a pictorial record of his incredible collection of shoes and boots.

Above
The Marie-Antoinette almost stole the show. The stately French queen sat majestically within her vitrine and gazed out from beneath her wig to the delight of our visitors, while Louis XIV looked on.

Right
The Marie-Antoinette is a style dear to Louboutin's heart. It shows the immense skill of French embroiderer Jean-François Lesage, who collaborated with Louboutin to create this shoe. Techniques include 'canetille', an embroidery stitch that figures on the head of Marie-Antoinette. The shoe also incorporates a 'Belle Poule', the French navy frigate that in 1778 defeated an English vessel.

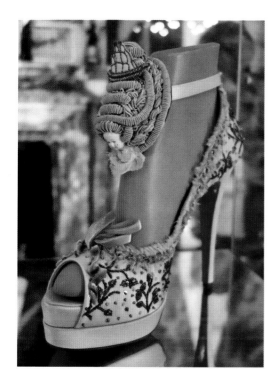

designed to look like Marie-Antoinette's head, complete with wig and galleons in full sail. The first Christian Louboutin shoe in a series of queens, the Marie-Antoinette, Queen of France, was perfect.

Arrangements were made to retrieve the Marie-Antoinettes from the archive and ship them to Blenheim. Alas, things do not always go according to plan and it was with growing dismay that I read this email just a few weeks before the exhibition was due to open:

We have located one pair of Marie-Antoinettes from the UK archive, however on arrival from storage...we found that only one foot remains in the storage box...We are reaching out to our Paris team to see if they can supply an alternative pair of the style – which should be no problem. Phew!

Louboutin certainly pulled out all the stops,

but unfortunately this email was followed by a good news/bad news phone call. Good news: a pair of Marie-Antoinettes had been sourced in Paris. Bad news: the distinctive fasteners that give the style its name were broken.

I need not have worried. We decided that having a single shoe on display would actually make a far greater impact and this was indeed the case. The Marie-Antoinette almost stole the show and, despite its glass display cloche being broken in transit, the stately French queen sat majestically within her vitrine and gazed out from beneath her wig at the admiring gazes of our visitors.

* * *

A footnote (pardon the pun). Imagine my dismay when I received the following email out of the blue, many months after the exhibition had finished and the Marie-Antoinette safely returned:

Hi Antonia
I hope you're well and trust the exhibition was a huge success.
May we please collect the Marie-Antoinette on Monday?

Thankfully, a few days later it was followed by:

I hope you had a lovely weekend.
Thank you so much for getting back to me. Apologies for alarming you, they are indeed here, they were just hidden away...!

A further footnote – as if one were not enough. Almost three years on, I am still waiting for a reply from Theresa May's office to my request to borrow a pair of those famous kitten-heeled shoes.

CHAPTER 11

Lady Diana: What's in a name?

'I never saw her wearing the dress…
then years later, there it was'

Designer Christina Stambolian on the 'Revenge Dress'

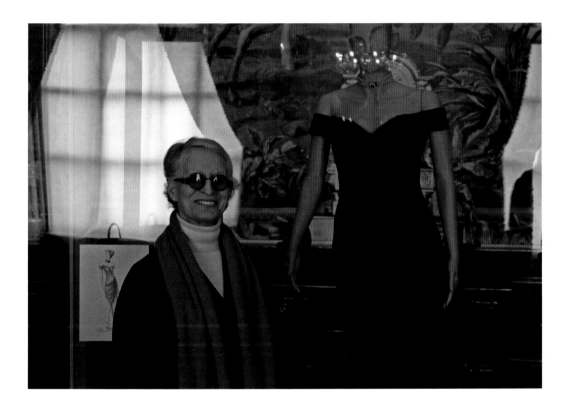

The year in which *A Passion for Fashion* made its appearance at Blenheim Palace – 2017 – was also, incredibly, the year that marked the twentieth anniversary of the death of Diana, Princess of Wales or, as I am sure many people will remember her, Lady Diana Spencer.

The Spencer-Churchill family at Blenheim Palace are distant cousins of the Spencer family at Althorp House in Northamptonshire – as previously mentioned – and to my knowledge the most recent 'Lady Di' was the fourth in the family to bear that name. She and the Dukes of Marlborough have a common ancestry dating back to the eighteenth century when Anne, a daughter of the 1st Duke and Duchess of Marlborough married into what one day would go on to become the late Princess of Wales's family.

When considering what to display in the Third State Room – the room that historically was the bedroom used by visiting royalty and heads of state – it seemed appropriate to include that year of all years a reference to Diana, Princess of Wales, and by association a look at what her two eighteenth-century Lady Diana Spencer ancestors would have been wearing, especially as they had been such interesting and forceful characters in the Palace's history.

To this end we had on display two eighteenth-century dresses that showed how fashions had changed somewhat sedately over the period of sixty years or so from the early 1720s to the late 1780s. The first Lady Diana (1710–1735) could have easily been seen in town wearing the elaborate green brocade silk

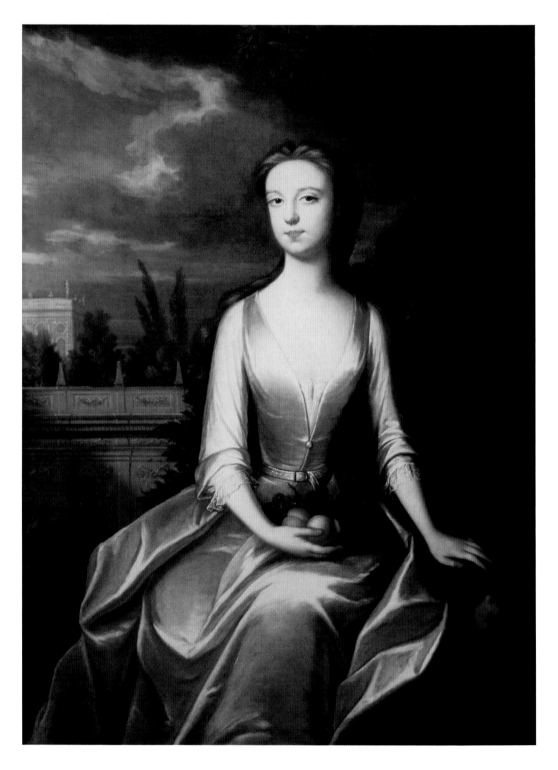

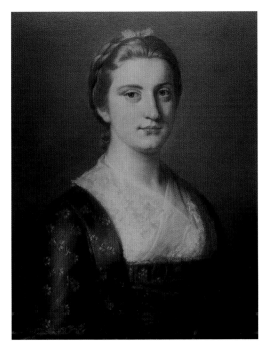

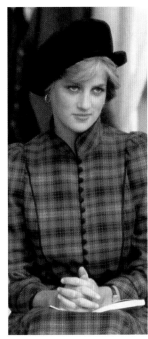

dress pictured later in this chapter.

The skirt of the dress – also known as an 'open robe' – was designed to part at the front, in order to display the elaborate design of the quilted petticoat beneath it. Quilted petticoats were popular throughout the eighteenth century and were worn not only to show off the exquisite sewing skills needed to create them, but also for warmth. The full skirt was pinned up at various points so that the hem of the petticoat was also on display, and the dress was worn with a 'handkerchief' around the neck and shoulders that served to protect the wearer's modesty during the day, as well as shielding her from the rays of the sun and from thus appearing like a coarsely tanned woman of the lower orders. The handkerchief would naturally be removed for evening wear.

Entries from the Blenheim ledgers of 1707

Previous page
I never saw her wearing the dress...and then years later, there it was'. Christina Stambolian in 2017 pictured at Blenheim Palace beside her most famous creation.

Left
Three Lady Diana Spencers. Three distinct styles. Three important and powerful women. *Portrait of Lady Diana Spencer, later Duchess of Bedford*, by Charles Jervas, 1722–31.

Above left
Diana Beauclerk, Self-portrait, date unknown.

Above right
Diana, Princess of Wales, at the Braemar Games, Scotland, 1981. Her 'tam-o'-shanter' is by the inimitable Stephen Jones.

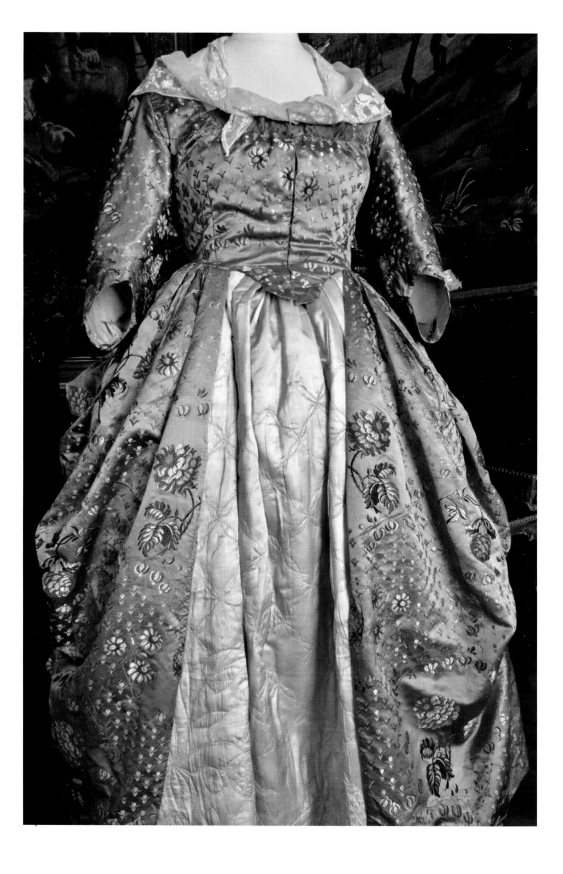

show a payment to an M. Reeves from the 1st Duchess of £4.10s.0d. (£4.50) for embroidering a long, green handkerchief with coloured silks and gold. This would be the equivalent of around £1,100 today,* so I think it is safe to assume that we are not talking about handkerchiefs as we currently know them. On a similar note, it is worth pointing out that the word 'skirt' was commonly used to describe the lower part of a gentleman's coat, while 'petticoat' referred to what we would today call a 'skirt'. Being aware of all this helps when trying to make sense of entries in a 300-year-old ledger.

The second of the eighteenth-century dresses in the Third State Room is of a style that would have been worn by Lady Diana Beauclerk (1734–1808). It is a silk, sack-back dress, a style that was popular from the mid to late part of the century. Its name refers to the two broad widths of silk on the back of the dress that fall in pleats down its entire length. This style began life as a comfortable, informal garment in the early 1700s that was worn in the home, before it developed into a fashionable day dress in the middle of the century and then ultimately, in the latter part of the century, into a formal dress worn only at court. Silk was originally used for such fashionable dresses until the very end of the 1700s, when printed linens and cottons also became popular.

Neither of these two dresses boasts integral pockets; instead, loose pockets were worn between the petticoats and the outer dress. Such pockets were invaluable accessories and served pretty much the same function as handbags do today. They were suspended from

*Bank of England inflation calculator

Left
An 'open robe' designed to part at the front in order to display the elaborate design of the quilted petticoat beneath it. Quilted petticoats were popular throughout the eighteenth century and were worn to show off the exquisite sewing skills needed to create them and also for warmth.

Above
A silk sack-back dress with two broad widths of silk at the back that fall in pleats down its entire length. This style began life as a comfortable, informal garment in the early 1700s that was worn in the home, before it developed into a fashionable day dress in the middle of the century and then ultimately, in the latter part of the century, into a formal dress worn only at court.

the waist and enabled a lady to have everything she needed to hand. The pockets were accessed via slits in the skirt of the dress that were designed for this purpose. The 1st Duchess of Marlborough had her pockets divided into four separate compartments so that she could organise everything exactly as she wished: her scissors, thimble, vinaigrette, snuffbox and, of course, two miniature portraits of the duke.

Unfortunately, the ties that suspended the pockets from the waist of the wearer could easily come undone and the pocket and its contents lost. This nursery rhyme appears on one level to make reference to just such an occurrence:

Lucy Locket lost her pocket
Kitty Fisher found it
Not a penny was there in it
Only ribbon 'round it!

It is only when we probe a little into its origins that we discover that Kitty Fisher was a famous eighteenth-century courtesan who is said to have taken up with a gentleman discarded by Lucy Locket, a barmaid, once he had spent all his money on her: hence the reference to an empty pocket. The ribbon in the rhyme was used to fasten the pocket not to the waist as a true lady would have done, but rather to the thigh as was the custom of the courtesan.

Dressmaking was regarded as a real skill and standards were incredibly high. The best dressmakers wasted barely a centimetre of fabric when cutting out a garment and they also had the aptitude to ensure that the finished dress would fit perfectly. The fabrics of the time tended to be heavily patterned and matching the design was an art in itself: a join had to be

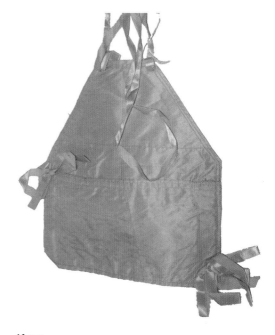

Above
Loose pockets were worn between the petticoats and the outer dress. They were invaluable accessories and served pretty much the same function as handbags do today.

The best dressmakers wasted barely a centimetre of fabric when cutting out a garment... the fabrics were heavily patterned - matching the design was an art in itself:

invisible from the right side of the fabric and only detectable on the reverse. It is no wonder that top dressmakers could command such high fees for their work. A ledger entry for 11 December 1707 records a payment of £15 for 'joyning silk for a manto & pettycoat': a considerable sum at a time when, on average, a laundry maid was paid £1 a month.

Fast forward now to the twentieth century and to the Lady Diana Spencer with whom we are all more familiar.

I thought about the hundreds of photographs I had seen of Diana and of the fashion leader she became, just like many royals before her. One of the two items of clothing that really stuck out in my mind, however, was her wedding dress: a fairy-tale dress.

Without further ado, I googled the name of the designer, Elizabeth Emanuel, and up popped both her website and her contact details. I promptly emailed this designer who had come to represent so many things and who, for me, epitomised a particular period in the history of the British monarchy. I could hardly believe it when she replied almost by return and asked me to give her a call 'anytime' for a chat. It was 4 March 2016, and this unremarkable Friday afternoon had suddenly become very remarkable indeed!

When Elizabeth and I spoke I explained the connection between Blenheim and the woman who had had such a great impact on her life. She was very positive about the idea of participating in a Blenheim-based exhibition on fashion and we arranged to meet. The day we met in Elizabeth's London studio is one that will stay with me for a long time. She answered the door in person and I was suddenly ever so slightly star-struck. This petite woman standing before me had sat and had coffee with one of the most famous women in the world and, over said coffee, had worked on creating probably the most famous wedding dress of the twentieth century: a far cry from the course of my normal working day.

Elizabeth chatted as she showed me her archive, which included photographs of her team of seamstresses working on the dress as they cut and stitched. She explained about the strict security that had to be put in place to keep the details of the dress away from the world's press, which involved her ordering a purpose-built safe that was so big it had to be brought in through the window of the Brook Street studio where the dress was made. The very fact that she and her husband David were the designers who had been commissioned to carry out this enviable task had to be hidden from even their closest friends and family.

Despite the relentless onslaught of social media, secrecy in such matters almost seems the norm now, especially with the recent weddings of Prince William and Prince Harry, but in 1981 all this media hype was new. Previous royal weddings had perhaps predictably relied on the excellent services of long-standing royal designers such as Norman Hartnell to create the bride's dress but this – like many things that Diana did – was a real departure from the norm.

Dotted around Elizabeth's studio were various trunks, each one a treasure trove. One of them housed the shoes that Diana had worn for her fittings, while another contained the actual dress pattern and, yet another, lace and sequined veiling, dress fabric and even partially sewn bodices and sleeves that, although they had been discarded in the making process, were

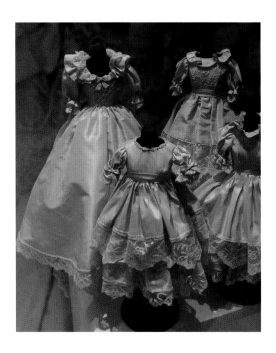

each a piece of fashion history. A further prize
was the scrapbook with its references, together
with sketches building up to the final design.

Elizabeth was incredibly generous with
her time and in agreeing to the loan of these
treasures but, as I said in the author's note,
things did not always go according to plan.
Originally, our exhibition was going to be
on for just four weeks. However, as plans
progressed and it became apparent that all of
the items on display, with the exception of Colin
Firth's breeches, were going to be loans, it was
decided that we could afford to extend it. Sadly,
because of other commitments, this meant
that Elizabeth's items would be on display
for only part of the exhibition's sixteen-week
duration, so eventually we had to make the
difficult decision not to include them at all. I
think this was the right thing to do, rather than
risk disappointing visitors who may have been

lured to Blenheim Palace with the promise of a
display by Elizabeth Emanuel, only to find there
was none!

So we fell back on plan B, which was…well, to
be honest there was no immediate plan B, but
thankfully that was soon to change.

I mentioned earlier that the wedding dress
was one of two of Diana's items of clothing that
stuck out in my mind. The other was a stunning
black dress, which was as different from her
wedding dress as it was possible to be: enter the
'Revenge Dress'.

On an autumn day in 1991, the Princess
of Wales arrived unannounced at the
Knightsbridge boutique of another young
designer. She was accompanied by her brother
Charles, the 9th Earl Spencer, and eventually
commissioned a stunning, black cocktail dress,
which Christina Stambolian designed and
made for her. The princess returned for fittings

and the finished dress was packaged, paid for and sent off to Kensington Palace. Christina did not see it again for almost three years.

In June 1994 the princess was due to fulfil a solo engagement at the Serpentine Gallery. The press reported that she would be wearing Valentino, but all that changed at the last moment and Diana appeared in the dress she had bought from Christina three years earlier. Until then, she had been apprehensive about wearing it in public as it was such a departure from her usual style. The effect was stunning, the message, at the end of her failed marriage, was clear and the dress itself was assured of a place in fashion history.

But how did the Revenge Dress make its way to Blenheim? Well, the truth is, it did not: I acquired its mate, the second of two that Christina had made. The original dress, worn and owned by Diana, was sold at auction for a reported $74,000. It has been put to good use in fundraising for the Scottish children's charity, Children 1st, and it is rather fitting to think that Diana's positive influence is still felt even after all these years.

So what of the other Revenge Dress? In the course of my research, the name of a vintage clothing specialist and auctioneer was mentioned to me, and so it was that I had the good fortune to come into contact with Kerry Taylor.

Kerry had sold the second Revenge Dress through her auction house, Kerry Taylor Auctions, and incredibly, given that we had yet to meet, she was kind enough to put me in touch with the gentleman who had bought this and many other items belonging, or related, to Diana (and to Audrey Hepburn as it happens, and Marilyn Monroe and Grace Kelly, to name

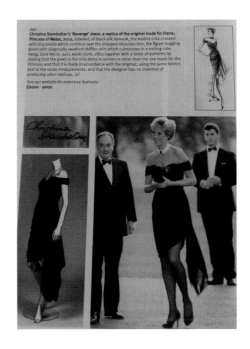

292
Christina Stambolian's 'Revenge' dress, a replica of the original made for Diana, Princess of Wales, 2010, labelled, of black silk damask, the bodice criss-crossed with tiny pleats which continue over the dropped shoulder-line, the figure-hugging gown with diagonally swathed chiffon skirt which culminates in a trailing side-swag, bust 86cm, 34in, waist 71cm, 28in; together with a letter of authenticity stating that the gown is the only dress in existence other than the one made for the Princess and that it is made in accordance with the original, using the same fabrics and to the same measurements, and that the designer has no intention of producing other replicas. (2)

See our website for extensive footnote.
£6000 - 9000

but a few). As a personal favour to Kerry – and what was fast becoming the norm for *A Passion for Fashion* – he agreed to loan us the dress.

In fact, Mr William Doyle, CEO of Newbridge Silverware, has his very own museum in Newbridge, Co. Kildare, which houses an immense collection of beautiful and sometimes quirky clothes. The museum has been built up over a relatively short period by William who bought the first item in the collection in 2006 and has never looked back.

Once *A Passion for Fashion* was up and running, William was kind enough to pay us a visit, along with his sister Pauline, Liz Farrell and Creative Director Simone Hassett-Costello. I was looking forward to meeting them all, but also slightly apprehensive: this was such an important and valuable exhibit (we had had to insure it for many times the £18,000 for which it was bought) and it really was irreplaceable. I hoped very much that they would be pleased with where we had placed it and how we had decided to display it.

I had many sleepless nights thinking about the head on the mannequin, which I have to be honest I disliked intensely, to the extent that I had wondered about taking a saw to it. In fact, there was a point when it appeared that the mannequin may have been too tall for the case that would be accommodating it for the next four months. Unfortunately, it just fitted with a couple of centimetres to spare and I must admit to having mixed feelings: a metal stump may have looked more stylish. You can be the judge of that.

I need not have worried. Pauline and Simone were with us for our opening reception and thanks in part to the time given and care shown to them by my colleague, Jo Young, they had a marvellous morning. They enjoyed the exhibition, but the thing that seemed to give them almost as much pleasure was being whisked around the Park by Jo in her nippy little mini, travelling to far-flung areas that visitors can normally only reach on foot.

A few weeks later, William and Liz also visited. They were in the UK for the opening of an exhibition of Diana's dresses at Kensington Palace to which William had loaned another of his pieces, Diana's engagement blouse, again by designers David and Elizabeth Emanuel. A small world.

I was slightly nervous about this visit too. Pauline and Simone had taken lots of photos of the dress when they saw it and were emailing them back to William as we walked through the Palace. He had declared himself to be happy with what he saw and I just hoped that the reality of seeing his beautiful dress in palatial

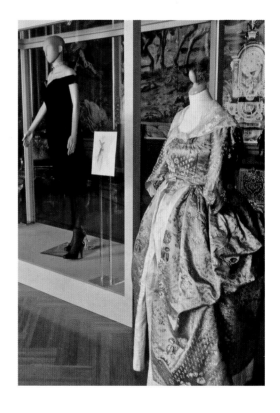

Above
Christina Stambolian's creation – an Italian silk jacquard and black silk chiffon cocktail dress – the exact copy of the one she made for Princess Diana – stands beside a late eighteenth-century dress in a style familiar to Diana Beauclerk, with its 'open robe' displaying the warm, quilted petticoat beneath it.

surroundings would not disappoint or dismay. Thankfully, he seemed genuinely pleased and amused to see that the dress had its very own case (thank you, Ashmolean Museum) and I think that having a piece from his collection in the home where Winston Churchill had been born was something that delighted him.

As we toured the Palace, I asked him how the CEO of a famous silverware company had come to be involved with frocks. Here is what happened. William had heard that the iconic black Givenchy dress worn by Audrey Hepburn in Breakfast at Tiffany's was due to be sold at auction by Christie's and, almost on a whim, decided that he would like to buy it. He had never been to a London auction before but, undeterred, he attended the sale. The lot came up, the room was tense and bidding began. The higher the bids went, the hotter under the collar he became, caught up in the frenzy of a bidding war. He was determined to win, right up until the moment when the bidding reached £650,000, and he realised that he was the underbidder to Givenchy, who would stop at almost nothing to acquire this particular dress for their collection, where they felt it rightfully belonged.

That particular dress evaded him, but needless to say, he did not come away empty-handed and he bought instead another little black dress worn by Audrey Hepburn, in the film *Charade*. The Irish press went to town and reported (incorrectly as it happened) that Mr Doyle had spent hundreds of thousands of euros on the Breakfast at Tiffany's dress: thousands of people marvelled at the news and travelled from far and wide to see this one dress.

A little while after this first purchase, William received a call from Beverly Hills-based Julien's Auctions, the leading auction house of celebrity memorabilia. The caller was the Executive Director of the auction house and an Irish ex-patriot, Martin J. Nolan. Mr Nolan understood that Mr Doyle had a museum and wondered if he would be interested in displaying the auction house's next lot: an amazing collection of Marilyn Monroe memorabilia including not only clothing, but also letters and original prints from iconic Monroe photo shoots?

Of course he would! Details were taken, dates arranged and the first thing William did when he came off the phone was to shout, 'Mick! Build me a museum!' This he did and a new star, the world-renowned Museum of Style Icons (MOSI), was born.

Back at Blenheim, we had the Revenge Dress, we had a beautiful case, Kate Ballenger, our tireless House Manager, had ensured that humidity and light levels would be perfect and the dress was set to become the focal point in one of the finest rooms in the Palace. However, I thought it would be rather nice if we could also include something of Christina Stambolian herself in the room in some way. Google came to my rescue once more and, having found Christina's website, I contacted her and we met up soon after. We had exchanged various emails and she had agreed to my displaying the design sketches for the dress alongside the dress itself. I had no real idea what she looked like – the images I had seen were slightly out of date – but, when it came to it, there could be no mistaking the striking woman with the quirky spectacles who stood in the foyer of the British Library and who greeted me with an enormous smile.

We sat and drank tea and chatted about how Diana's purchase of the dress had come about.

Essentially, it was all very simple.

Christina had hoped that Diana might approach her, as she had done a number of other British-based designers, and one day in the autumn of 1991 she did, unannounced. She and her brother Charles visited Christina's boutique in Beauchamp Place. The princess was looking for a cocktail dress for a special occasion. Diana and Christina considered various items in the boutique. Diana was an easy person to be around and she inspired Christina, who had already thought about the sort of thing she might create for Diana if the opportunity arose. Together they discussed various ideas and eventually Diana asked her brother for his opinion on the design that Christina had come up with: he was, understandably, happy to trust to his sister's good taste.

The dress was commissioned and the process began. However, Diana did not leave the boutique empty-handed, but with two blouses and a second dress.

Christina recalled that as she had not come across any reports or photos of Diana wearing her dress, she had put the whole thing to the back of her mind, until the day in June 1994 when the world's press went mad. Suddenly, Christina's name was on everyone's lips as the designer of a most remarkable dress worn by a most remarkable woman.

Interestingly, Christina dislikes the term 'Revenge Dress', as that had not been the creative force behind the fabulous Italian silk jacquard and black silk chiffon cocktail dress. The idea had been simply to create something specifically for Diana, a natural progression from the distinctive designs in the boutique that already bore the marks of Christina's own unique style.

Right
Christina's sketch for the front of the 'Revenge Dress'.

Below
Christina's sketch for the back of the 'Revenge Dress'.

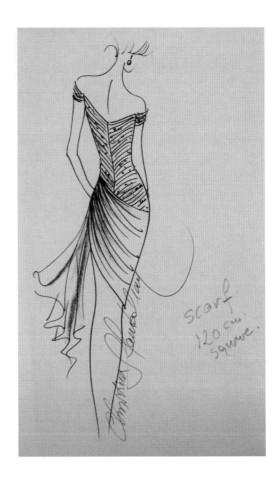

Over twenty years later, Christina still has mixed feelings about the whole experience. Her memories of Diana at that first meeting are of someone with grace and presence, friendly, kind and with a great sense of humour: qualities not easily forgotten. There were other positives, too. She met some wonderful people, including, of course, Diana, and others who were perhaps not as sincere. She had some fabulous experiences, such as meeting Diana again, at the press launch of the charity auction in which many of the princess's dresses, including the Revenge Dress, were being sold. Diana joked that she would have a bit of trouble squeezing into Christina's dress all those years later. Christina will always have the great satisfaction of knowing that this stunning little black dress, which started out as a daring idea in her Kensington boutique, is not only used in charity work, but also continues to be recognised and spoken of the world over.

When we had finished chatting, Christina produced from the depths of her bag a number of sketches and asked me to choose which ones I would like to take with me. I almost choked on my tea: I had not come prepared to take these treasures back with me that same day.

Christina was extraordinarily generous on our first meeting and has continued to be so ever since. I declined her offer of taking the sketches with me there and then, but explained that I wanted to make sure that they were fully insured and correctly packaged before they left her possession: I had visions of being hit by a bus on my way home! The result: two of her exquisite sketches – the front of the dress and the back – on display beside THAT dress, and a friendship that I hope will endure for years to come.

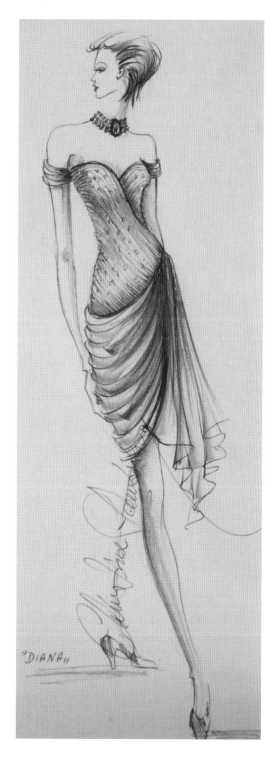

"DIANA"

CHAPTER 12

Christian Dior: Quite a Revolution

'I adore the English, dressed not only in the tweeds which suit them so well, but also in those flowing dresses in subtle colours.'

—Christian Dior

If I were given the opportunity of meeting any member of the Marlborough family who has slept beneath the vast roof of Blenheim Palace over the past eleven generations, I would be torn between Sarah, the 1st Duchess, and Mary, the 10th Duchess. I would be rather trepidatious in either case: both of them had reputations for being rather strong-willed and for not suffering fools gladly, but I think that eventually I would have to come down in favour of meeting Duchess Mary.

Alexandra Mary Hilda Cadogan was born on 22 February 1900, one of the six children (five of them girls) of Henry Cadogan, Viscount Chelsea, and his wife, the Honourable Mildred Sturt. She married 'Bert', the 10th Duke of Marlborough, in 1920, when she was just a few days short of her twentieth birthday, in a ceremony in St Margaret's, Westminster. The wedding was attended by the king and queen and other royals, as well as by Lady Randolph Churchill, her son, Winston, and his wife Clementine. It was almost twelve years since Winston Churchill had cut such a poorly dressed figure at his own wedding in the very same church.

Early photographs of the young Mary show a handsome, strong-jawed woman, fashionably dressed and coiffed, with determination etched in her features. She would need that determination years later, when at thirty-four years old she became the 10th Duchess and took on the rather formidable task of turning Blenheim into a home for her husband and growing family. Moving into a Palace that boasted just one bathroom was hardly ideal; add to that the pressure of safeguarding not only her family and staff, but also Blenheim itself, during the Second World War and I am

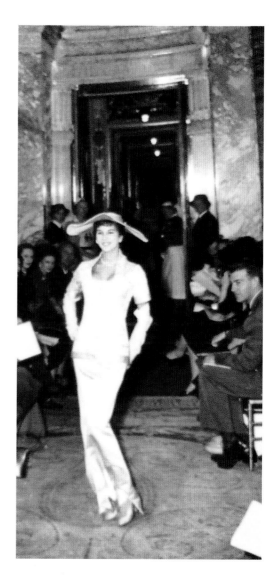

Above
Christian Dior's 1954 show was held to raise funds for the Red Cross. It was the first collection to be presented in a British stately home

'Simplicity, good taste and grooming are the three fundamentals of good dressing and these do not cost money.'

—*Christian Dior*

sure you will begin to see what I mean.

For most of her too short life – she died a few months after her sixty-first birthday – the duchess was a passionate supporter of the British Red Cross Society. During the First World War she had nursed as a VAD (Voluntary Aid Detachment) in a London hospital and then in the Second World War she helped to administer the eight Red Cross auxiliary hospitals in Oxfordshire. Despite all this, and looking after her own expanding family, the duchess also made time to find temporary accommodation in the area for the many relatives from all over the country, who were visiting their loved ones in local hospitals.

Duchess Mary became President of the local Oxford branch of the Red Cross and in 1954 she hit upon a marvellous way of continuing to raise funds for this important charity. She decided against the more usual fundraising methods – jumble sales, the occasional whist drive, etc. – and chose instead to host a fashion show. She obviously had a flair for fashion and style and in 1958 had even designed a new uniform for women members of the Red Cross. Her creation replaced the previous military-style uniform with a far more feminine and businesslike navy blue suit.

The duchess herself was not a patron of the relatively new House of Dior; she preferred to use British designers such as Hardy Amies to dress herself and her daughters for formal occasions. She was also fortunate in being able to enlist her American mother-in-law, Consuelo Balsan (née Vanderbilt), for help in obtaining clothes for said daughters while clothes rationing was still in force in the UK. Clothes rationing was finally discontinued in March 1949, two years after Dior first established his label in Paris, amid much hoo-ha about the amount of fabric used in his creations at that time of continuing austerity.

Christian Dior took the fashion world by storm with his 'New Look': so named because of a chance comment by Carmel Snow, Editor-in-Chief of *Harper's Bazaar*, who, at the end of Dior's debut fashion show in February 1947, exclaimed with pleasure, 'It's quite a revolution, dear Christian! Your dresses have such a new look!' A correspondent from Reuters overheard the conversation and quickly wrote it down and sent it by courier back to the US. And so it was that the citizens of America heard the term even before it was reported in France. After the many bleak, grey war years, Dior's wonderful clothes in rich colours and fabrics together with their distinctive new styling were like a breath of fresh air.

Dior, like the 10th Duchess, was a passionate supporter of the Red Cross. The opportunity to present a collection in a British stately home for the very first time resulted in the historic fashion show that took place on 3 November 1954. Dior's Paris Winter Collection – the H-Line (H for 'haricot vert' or green bean) – was generally well received with its lengthened torsos and unbroken waistlines, as was the chance to win one of his creations for the price of a £1 raffle ticket.

The show took a great deal of organisation. Duchess Mary, dressed in her Red Cross uniform, travelled to Paris to meet Christian Dior. He made a return visit to Blenheim and declared himself to be satisfied with the proposed setting for his creations. It could not fail, especially given Dior's penchant for all things British; here was a Frenchman who wore suits tailored on Savile Row and drew inspiration from English and Scottish checks and tweeds.

The duchess was an excellent organiser and administrator and also extraordinarily well connected. Once the concept of having a fashion show at Blenheim became a reality, she called upon her many friends and

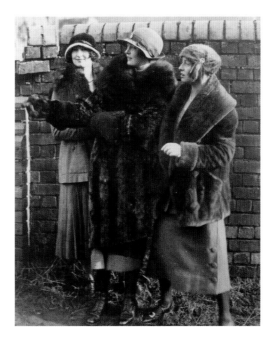

Above
The 10th Duchess of Marlborough (centre) as a twenty-one-year-old. By the time this photograph was taken she had become a dedicated supporter of the Red Cross, having worked as a VAD during the First World War. She eventually became President of her local Oxford branch until her death in 1961.

Below
The duchess's invitation to buy tickets to the 1954 Dior Fashion Show. She called upon her many friends and acquaintances and wrote to each of them asking that they support her plan by purchasing tickets priced at five guineas each (£5.25). However, as most of the 'guests' had paid to be at Blenheim, rather than being there as individual guests of the Marlboroughs, the duke and duchess, did not 'personally receive them'.

Her Royal Highness Princess Margaret has graciously consented to give her patronage to a showing of Monsieur Christian Dior's Paris Winter Collection on November 3rd, 1954, at Blenheim Palace, which their Graces The Duke and Duchess of Marlborough have kindly lent for the purpose.

The Duke and Duchess of Marlborough extend their hospitality on this occasion for the benefit of the British Red Cross Society, of which the Duchess is a member of the Council. The presentation will take place under the personal supervision of Monsieur Christian Dior who, as a contribution to the Red Cross, is lending his French collection which will be presented by all his Paris Mannequins.

Blenheim Palace has entertained the most illustrious men and women and the greatest artists and master designers of the last two centuries. Here you will have the opportunity of attending a unique occasion which has not been rivalled even in the halcyon days of this most noble house.

An application form is enclosed for your easy convenience. Tickets, five guineas each. The number of seats is limited and those wishing to attend are asked to make early application.

The Palace will be open from 2.30 p.m. to guests attending the function.

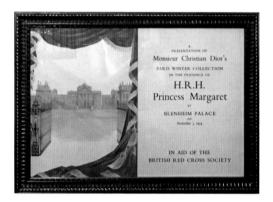

acquaintances and wrote to each of them
asking that they support her plan by purchasing
tickets priced at five guineas each (£5.25). It
made me smile, however, to read a report in
the local paper, the *Oxford Mail*, which states
that, as most of the 'guests' had paid to be at
Blenheim, rather than being there as individual
guests of the Marlboroughs, the duke and
duchess would not 'personally receive them'.
Standards had to be maintained!

Friends living locally were called upon to
provide accommodation for the mannequins
and various members of the entourage. Family
friend Willie Freud was among those to lend
his continued support. He had previously been
prevailed upon to help move furniture out
of the Palace's State Rooms when pupils and
staff of Malvern College were evacuated there
during the war. He now rose to the occasion
by playing host to mannequins Simone and
Claire. HRH The Princess Margaret, another
family friend – particularly of the duchess's
youngest daughter, Lady Rosemary Muir (née
Spencer-Churchill) – was guest of honour. She

was already a patron of Maison Dior and was
famously photographed by Cecil Beaton on the
occasion of her twenty-first birthday in 1951,
wearing a magnificent one-shouldered, cream
Dior couture gown that showed her – and her
54-cm waist – off to perfection.

Despite her close friendship with Princess
Margaret, Lady Rosemary did not attend this
particular show. She had been married the
previous year – a few weeks after acting as
one of the Maids of Honour at the coronation
of Princess Margaret's older sister – and was
by now heavily pregnant with her first child
who was born just four days after the show.
Different times...or was it an attempt to avoid a
repetition of the circumstances of the birth of
her distant cousin, Winston Churchill?*

Almost everything went according to plan:
3,000 champagne saucers were ordered
from Paris and duly arrived and Blenheim

*Winston Churchill had been born two months prematurely
on 30 November 1874 while his parents were attending a St
Andrew's Day Ball, which, just like the fashion show, was taking
place in the Long Library.

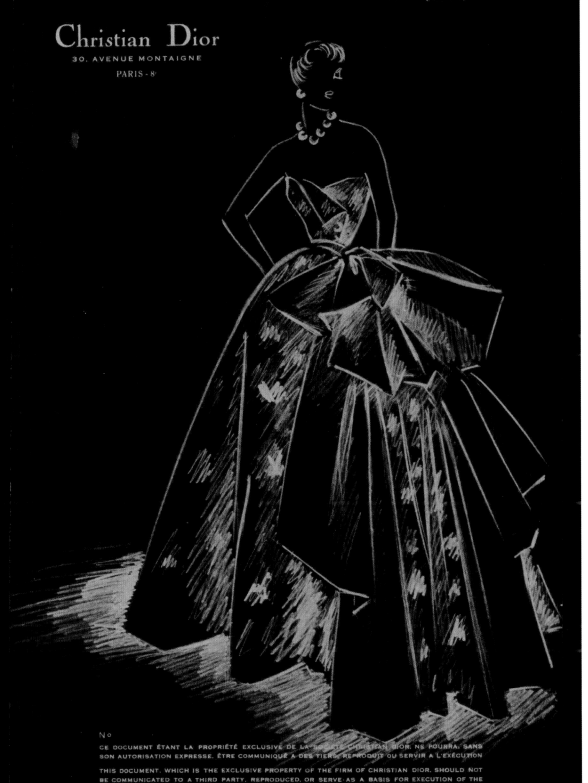

MARGARET

Christian Dior
30, AVENUE MONTAIGNE
PARIS - 8e

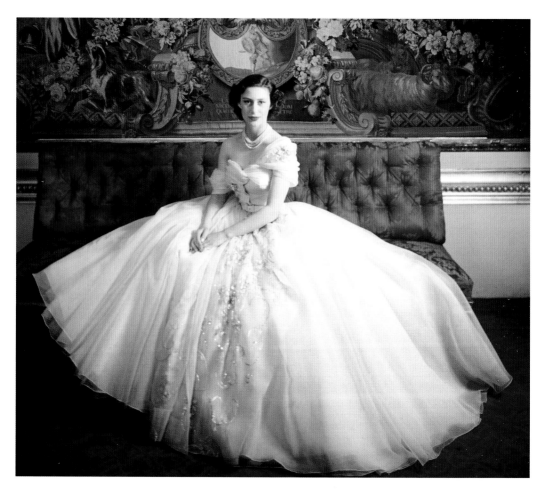

Above
Princess Margaret
photographed by Cecil
Beaton at Buckingham
Palace in 1951 wearing her
iconic Dior gown.

Right
The duchess, seated beside
Christian Dior, inspects
part of the collection. She
was determined that things
would run smoothly and
even helped to iron some of
the frocks prior to the 1954
show.

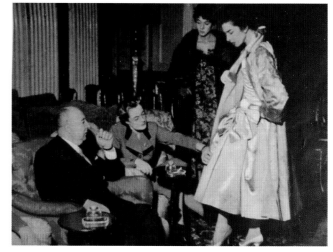

Right
Palace Administrator
Archie Illingworth enjoys
a moment with a Dior
mannequin in 1954. Archie
was at the helm when the
Palace first opened its
doors to the public. It is
unlikely that his Palace
equivalent today would be
enjoying a quiet smoke and
a glass of champagne in
similar circumstances.

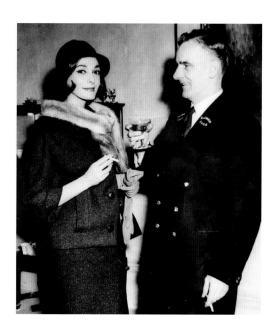

staff spent the weekend preparing for the show. Life was easier in those days, when the Palace was only open for a few half days a week – and hardly at all during the shoot season – a far cry from the 364 days a year that the Palace is open to the public today. The resident electrical engineer – creator of the most splendid centrepieces for the Blenheim Christmas table – was commandeered to install additional floodlights: bright enough to light the collection, but not so bright that the audience would be dazzled by them. Chairs – 2,000 of them – were acquired and set out and the eve of the show arrived, but sadly not the mannequins.

The Dior party was late leaving London Airport, so the rehearsal planned for the eve of the show was postponed until noon on the actual day. However, they arrived at Blenheim in time to enjoy a buffet supper at the champagne reception held for them in the Great Hall and tucked into chicken, hams, game and fruit before being whisked off to their host families.

The big day finally arrived, the postponed rehearsal took place and the mannequins familiarised themselves with the route through the State Rooms. This started at the Coral Rooms (now the Operations Office), continued through the Long Library and the State Rooms and finally into the Grand Cabinet on the private side of the Palace.

Their hair was dressed by Keith Hall and a team of stylists from his Nottingham salon. Keith, a friend of the Duchess of Devonshire, had travelled to France in the period immediately after the Second World War to learn about hairdressing. His mentor was Alexandre de Paris, the coiffeur whose name was synonymous with French chic and elegance, and favourite not only of Dior, but also of Coco Chanel, Yves Saint-Laurent, Jean-

Paul Gaultier and many more. It was probably through his connection to both Alexandre (Louis Alexandre Raimond) and the Duchess of Devonshire – a friend of Duchess Mary – that Keith Hall's services were secured for the show. Hairdressing was clearly in his genes and today his grandson, Andrew Hall, is a director of a leading group of hairdressing salons in Oxfordshire.

Ticket holders had been asked to take their seats by 3.45pm, although on this auspicious occasion they had been allowed to enter the Palace for over an hour prior to that in order to view its treasures and soak up the atmosphere. Princess Margaret, who had travelled by train to Oxford, was met by the duke in his chauffeur-driven car and arrived at Blenheim just before 4.00pm, when the two-hour show was scheduled to start. After inspecting a guard of honour by the Red Cross, the Princess took her seat on a red damask armchair in the centre of the Long Library beneath the

watchful gaze of a marble bust of the 1st Duke. The fourteen mannequins were splendid and it was calculated that during the exhausting show each of them would have walked almost 5 km through the nine State Rooms.

The Long Library alone is 55 m long and the second longest room in any private house in the country; the longest is at Castle Howard, John Vanbrugh's other monumental creation. It is the most calming of rooms with its peach-coloured walls and exquisite carvings. It must have witnessed many interesting events in the hundreds of years since it was built: ladies promenading, Anthony van Dyck's equestrian portrait of the ill-fated Charles I being taken down, the installation of the fabulous Willis Organ, weary soldiers convalescing during the First World War, schoolboys sleeping and getting up to mischief during the the the Second World War, and even an invasion by MI5 during the latter years of that same war once the boys had left. The arrival of Dior must have

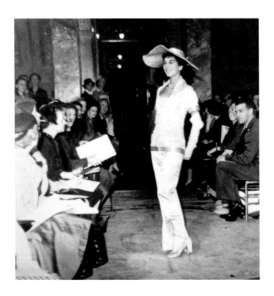

Left
Amadis on show in 1954, with hairstylist Keith Hall (seated right) looking on. It was probably through his connection to both French coiffeur Alexandre de Paris and the Duchess of Devonshire – a friend of Duchess Mary – that Hall's services were secured for the show. Hairdressing was clearly in his genes and today his grandson, Andrew Hall, is a director of a leading group of hairdressing salons in Oxfordshire.

Right
Princess Margaret sits back and enjoys the 1954 show. The 10th Duke and Duchess of Marlborough are seated either side of her. The duke enjoys a joke with one of his friends who provided accommodation for one of Dior's mannequins.

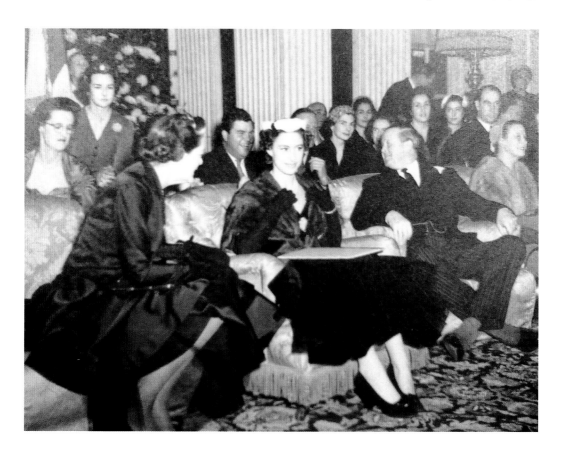

been a welcome respite.

For the show, the format adopted by Dior at Blenheim was identical to that used when presenting clothes at Maison Dior in Paris. A 'barker' would announce the name of each dress: 'Amadis, ensemble de soir, Aminte, ensemble déjeuner-dîner' and then alphabetically right through to ensemble number 110, 'Zulma, ensemble fin de journée', until finally two specials, Cortége and Blenheim, both described simply as 'robe'. In 1954, the role of barker fell to Red Cross member, Mrs Madeleine Stratton.

As each style was called, the mannequin would walk graciously through the State Rooms: there was no catwalk. Each dress was made especially for the mannequin and corseted so that she would assume the shape required by Dior. The making process could take up to six weeks and the final fitting was overseen by Dior himself; he disliked touching the models and instead would prod them with a stick. The corsets – just as the ones worn by women a century before – could be rather uncomfortable and prevented the wearer from being able to sit or do very little else, other than to raise an arm to hold a glass of champagne: thank Heaven!

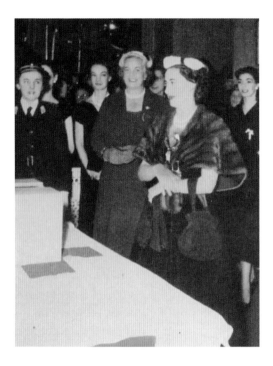

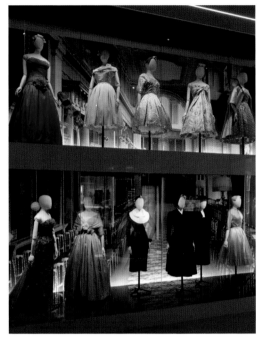

Once the whole collection had been presented with great style and grace, all that remained was for Princess Margaret to pick the winning ticket from the raffle, which she had consented to do at approximately 7.00pm. It was rather an anticlimax to discover that the owner of winning ticket number 754, a Mr Watson of Haslemere in Surrey, had already left for home and, despite all of our best efforts, we have not been able to find a record in Dior's archive of the woman who eventually had the pleasure of receiving one of these timeless outfits made especially for her.

There were approximately 2,000 guests at the show. Its financial success was assured and the duchess was able to present the Red Cross with a cheque for £8,110.8s.10d.: the equivalent of over £200,000 today.*

This groundbreaking show received a huge amount of press coverage: sixty members of the press had been invited to attend and it was a great success. The only person to be left a little disappointed by the afternoon was Dior himself because, mindful of the good that could be done by publicity, no French photographers had been invited.

The 1954 show was such a success at raising much-needed money for the Red Cross that the duchess was persuaded to arrange a second fundraiser, planned for 12 November 1958. Sadly, Christian Dior had died in the previous October, just ten years after he had founded his famous fashion house. This time, the shy twenty-two-year-old Yves St Laurent, who was by now Dior's top designer, was at the helm and travelled to Blenheim to supervise the event. The value of the dresses to be modelled was put at £111,000: the equivalent

Far left

Princess Margaret prepares to draw the winning raffle ticket. It was rather an anticlimax to discover that the owner of winning ticket number 754, a Mr Watson of Haslemere in Surrey, had already left for home and, despite our best efforts, we have not been able to find a record in Dior's archive of the woman who eventually had the pleasure of receiving one of these timeless outfits made especially for her.

Left

The Dior in Britain case at the V&A's *'Dior Designer of Dreams'* exhibition 2019. The Long Library at Blenheim - complete with catwalk from the 2016 show - forms the backdrop for these wonderful vintage Dior outfits

Right

Princess Margaret congratulates Yves St Laurent in 1958. Dior had died the previous year and the shy twenty-two-year-old was now Maison Dior's top designer.

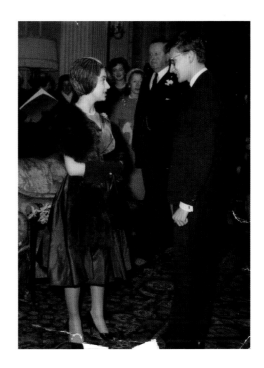

of £2.5 million today.*

At the 1958 show, as at the earlier one, there were around 2,000 guests, most of them women, to enjoy the parade of 136 dresses that made up Maison Dior's Paris Winter Collection. According to newspaper reports, things started rather slowly and the audience seemed in complete awe of both dresses and mannequins. This did not last, however, and once Princess Margaret – guest of honour for the second time – relaxed with a cigarette to enjoy the spectacle (imagine doing that today) the audience seemed to relax with her and the tension evaporated. This time, Lady Rosemary was able to attend. The beautiful, tall, slender twenty-nine-year-old had actually been asked at the outset to model some of the gowns, but

unfortunately she had to refuse this unique opportunity as, by now, she was pregnant with her second child. This was a time when expectant mothers were clearly not supposed to draw attention to themselves.

Preparations were just as intense and prolonged for the second show as for the first, but made easier by previous experience. The day was not without the occasional mishap, however. The most indisposed of all was a reporter with indigestion: a result of too many tasty pre-show canapés perhaps? Princess Margaret was almost required to exit Oxford station by the same route as the general public, a calamity prevented by someone tracing a mislaid key. A programme was knocked from the hand of a guest by an over-enthusiastic flourish of a mannequin's stole, and a lady in the audience, easing her foot from a too tight

*Bank of England inflation calculator

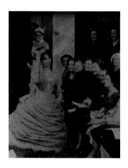

Left
In 1954 the beautiful, smiling Victoire Doutreleau, with her 48-cm waist, nearly lost her hat when modelling the shocking pink Zépherine; however, she quickly tugged Simone Mirman's creation from her head without faltering and continued on her way.

Right
Models parade through the Long Library on 31 May 2016 for the launch of Christian Dior's S/S17 Cruise Collection. The whole show, after months of preparation, lasted only twelve minutes.

shoe, was alarmed to see the shoe carried off as it caught on a coat being trailed stylishly behind another mannequin. It could have been far worse.

The beautiful, smiling Victoire Doutreleau, with her 48-cm waist, nearly lost her hat when modelling the shocking pink (recently rediscovered Zépherine); however, she quickly tugged Simone Mirman's creation from her head without faltering and continued on her way. It is fascinating to note when looking at the photographs of the show that the majority of the women present, including the mannequins, are wearing hats. The only exceptions are the duchess and her two daughters who were, of course, at home.

Fast forward fifty-eight years and Dior returned to Blenheim Palace for a third time. There had been talk of it for many years and other fundraising fashion shows had taken place in between times: notably in the mid-1970s, given by Oxford Campus. The beneficiary was to be Sobell House, a local hospice, and the clothes being modelled were complemented by a fabulous display of award-winning costumes by Jane Robinson, which were designed for the 1974 Thames Television, Jennie: Lady Randolph Churchill, and worn by

Lee Remick in the title role.

When plans and arrangements were finally agreed after much discussion and negotiation, Maison Dior launched its Prêt-à-Porter Collection Cruise 2017 by Lucie Meier and Serge Ruffieux, at Blenheim Palace on 31 May 2016, amid much excitement and anticipation, and that was just the Blenheim staff.

The Palace was closed to visitors for two days while everything was set up: chairs and programmes laid out, flowers and food arranged, champagne chilled and, unlike the previous shows, a hand-painted, Blenheim-inspired catwalk laid. The route through the State Rooms was exactly the same as that taken by those elegant, smiling 1950s' mannequins, but there the similarity ended.

There were no 'barkers' this time, just a programme listing the fifty-five outfits shown by the fifty-five models. There were short descriptions for the clothes rather than exotic names: 'Manteau en laine écrue' or 'Robe en satin de soie jaune', which became 'Ecru wool coat' and 'Yellow silk satin dress' for those less linguistically able or romantically inclined. The gentle 1950s' music from the Willis Organ was replaced by pounding garage music, spotlights blazed and dazzled, and the smiles

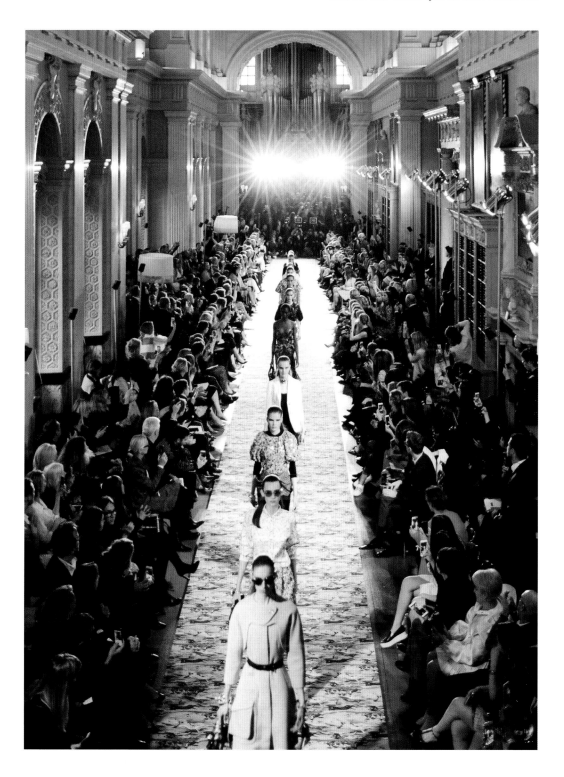

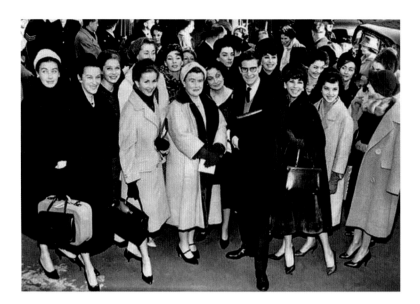

Left
Yves St Laurent with
mannequins: Svetlana
Lloyd is second on the
right. Svetlana had been
one of the mannequins who
visited in 1958 to show off
the latest creations of Yves
St Laurent and returned
for the 2016 show.

of Victoire, Simone and Lucky were exchanged for the studious frowns of Dior's current stable of models.

The celebrity audience had been transported from London to Oxfordshire on the specially chartered Orient Express, and then chauffeured by a fleet of limousines to Blenheim Palace where a fanfare of trumpets greeted them in the pouring rain. Among the hundreds of celebrities was a very notable guest, Svetlana Lloyd, and it was certainly not her first visit to Blenheim Palace: she had been one of the mannequins who took part in the 1958 show of Yves St Laurent's latest creations.

While most members of the Blenheim staff were not allowed inside the Palace on the day of the Cruise launch, a small number were required to be at hand and the dress code was strictly black and white. One colleague who favoured more brightly coloured clothes was advised that she might be more comfortable working from home on that particular day!

Luckily, I was able to plead my case to be present at the show, as I had built up a virtual relationship with the amazing Soïzic Pfaff, Directrice Dior Héritage. Over the months leading up to the Cruise launch, we had been in regular contact and I had furnished her with information and images from the earlier Blenheim shows. In exchange, she took me on a personal tour of the dresses and artefacts that had travelled from her archive in Paris to be displayed in the Great Hall: a fantastic tribute to the fashion shows of the 1950s and something rather special for the 2016 audience to see.

When it was time for the show to start, I positioned myself in the Long Library where I remained hidden behind the immense statue of Queen Anne. I was with Amber Carter, a much younger colleague, and not being terribly au fait with current celebrity, I asked her if she had spotted anyone famous. The only name that sprang to her mind was Bella Hadid, who was walking that day: such an interesting term.

The show itself began fashionably late. Family members sat beneath the marble bust

bust of the 1st Duke, just as they had been in the previous shows, the models marched grim-faced through the State Rooms...and the whole thing was over in twelve minutes flat. It brought to my mind a meeting I had had with Caroline Issa earlier in the year at Bicester Village where she and I had been 'in conversation'. She is the fashion editor of *Tank* magazine and on some days she attends one show after another, all of them of similar length to the one we had just witnessed. How they do not all blur into one is a mystery.

The show generated much news coverage the following day, both via social media and more traditional means, and part way through the morning I received an email from my daughter with a link to some of the reports and a message that read, 'Mum, you were with some really cool people yesterday.' When I followed the link I came across many names I recognised and outfits I recalled: Bianca Jagger, Eva

---

'Mr Dior did not touch the models, but gently touched [us] with a stick to let others in the room see what he meant'

—*Svetlana Lloyd, model at Christian Dior from 1956 to 1958 (St Laurent)*

Herzigová, Stephen Jones, Kate Beckinsale, Alexa Chung and Princess Diana's niece, Lady Kitty Spencer, to name but a few. I had been aware of what they were wearing, but anything else had passed me by.

Lady Rosemary was in the audience once more – sadly the only surviving family member who had attended one of the previous Dior shows – and she was accompanied by her nieces and nephews. I am sure that the Marlborough party found the spectacle of interest, but if they had expected the elegance and chic of the 1950s' Dior show, then they were probably disappointed.

How best to illustrate the Dior connection in our *A Passion for Fashion* exhibition? I remembered once seeing a striking black and white dress at the local museum in Woodstock and discovered that it was part of the collection of a museum in Coventry: the Herbert Art Gallery & Museum. Enter curator Ali Wells, who agreed that we could have the dress for our exhibition, but pointed out that it was possibly 'in the style of' Dior rather than by the great man himself. As though the loan of the black and white dress were not helpful enough, however, she was also responsible for the loan of the four late Victorian outfits on display in the First State Room, which typified Consuelo's daily wardrobe, as well as assorted crinolines, garters and even a 1950s' girdle.

Another stroke of luck came in the shape of BBC One's *Antiques Roadshow* of all things. An episode in October 2016 featured a stunning orange dress, definitely by Dior, complete with original box and labels. That week, the show had been broadcast from Broughton Castle, a stone's throw from Blenheim, as hopefully would be its owner.

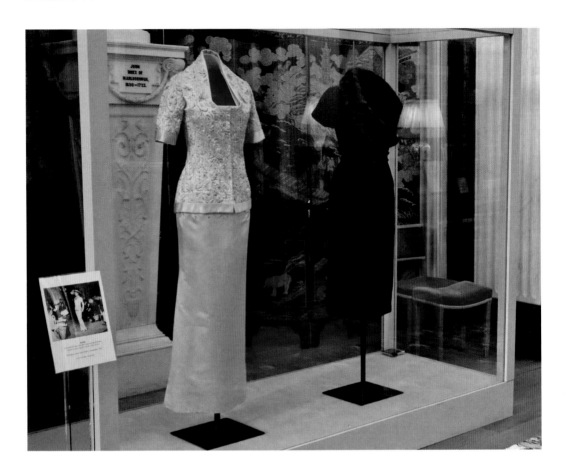

Without further ado, I contacted the BBC and asked them to pass on my contact details to the owner of the dress and explained my interest. Then I held my breath and waited. But I did not have to wait too long and one autumn day Cheryl Burgess arrived at Blenheim, complete with the Dior dress that had belonged to her mother for me to look at. And, yes, she would be willing to let us include it in our display. What luck!

I would have liked to include something from the Cruise collection in the Dior display, but time was running out. Necessity is the mother of invention, so instead two life-sized, free-

Above
Back at Blenheim: Amadis and Mazette. Each gown came complete with its own bespoke mannequin, which fitted it perfectly: it was even painted the same colour as its dress so that it would not detract from the beauty of the gown itself.

standing cut-outs of the 2016 models were commissioned and were placed on pieces of the Blenheim catwalk that formed part of our Dior display in the Long Library.

Given that Dior had been such an important part of Blenheim's fashion history, one Dior dress and one beautiful, but 'in the style of', Dior dress did not seem to me to be enough of a display. Our budget had virtually run out and I was bemoaning this situation to my long-suffering husband who, sensibly it turned out, suggested that I might look for sponsorship.

Enter Bicester Village...

By now it was December 2016 and *A Passion for Fashion* was due to open in two months' time. Sophie Hedley and Bicester Village really did come up trumps. Working in the heritage sector is incredibly rewarding, but finances, or lack of them, impose a continual restraint. Thankfully, this does not seem to be the case in the high-end retail sector. The generous sponsorship we received from Bicester Village meant that not only did we double our original budget for the exhibition, but also that we would be able to afford to transport and display two Dior dresses that had originally been shown at the 1954 fashion show.

Enter Amadis and Mazette, the latter – along with the original Bar Suit – being a personal favourite. A member of Soïzic's team, travelled from Avenue Montaigne to install these two exquisite gowns. They arrived in large metal cases – just as they had done in the 1950s – and were beautifully wrapped in layers of protective tissue. Each came complete with its own bespoke mannequin, which fitted it perfectly: it was even painted the same colour as its dress so that it would not detract from the beauty of the gown itself.

Sophie and other members of the Bicester Village team came and watched the installation take place and had a sneak preview of the exhibition, which was due to open a couple of days later. They were, I think, happy with what they had lent their name to.

With the help of Christina, another of my colleagues who had kindly offered their help, the installation was completed quickly and efficiently and the possibility of the person from Dior catching an earlier train back to Paris became a reality. Enter Jo and her mini again. She took him to where she was parked in Kennel Courtyard and off they went, only to be engulfed by that most English of things: a hunt, complete with hounds. I do not know how Jo managed to negotiate horses, hounds and riders, but she did get to the station with moments to spare and so this particular entente cordiale remains intact and, thankfully, the Dior display with its dresses, catwalk and memorabilia, past and present, became a success.

A footnote to all this was the magnificent aptly named *Couturier du Rêve* exhibition at the Musée des Arts Décoratifs in Paris. This 'designer of dreams' initiative was put together to celebrate seventy years of Maison Dior and it certainly achieved its aim. It was something I desperately wanted to see, particularly Dior's early work, and time was running out. And so it was that one cold November morning in 2017 found me and two of my daughters aboard a very early Eurostar bound for Paris. I had been in touch with Soïzic and asked if we might meet for coffee at some stage during our visit. She said she would be delighted, but I have to say that, as it turned out, her hospitality and that of her team surpassed all expectation.

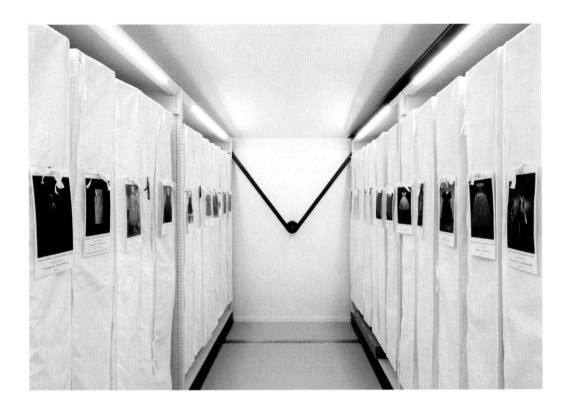

We were met outside the museum by Hélène Starkman (who, at the time of writing, was involved with the 2019 Dior exhibition at the V&A) and having deftly circumnavigated the crowds waiting to be let in, we spent the next couple of hours touring the exhibition in Hélène's knowledgeable and most congenial company. As though that were not enough, we were then whisked off to One Dior, Avenue Montaigne – just opposite the original Dior couture house – to view the heritage centre and to meet up with Soïzic.

The heritage centre is exceptional: the archive had not, as is so often the case, been of high priority and in some areas had glaring omissions, but now it was receiving the attention it deserved. It had been moved from the original ateliers at 30 Avenue Montaigne into a purpose-built centre, ready to welcome the international interest that Dior knew the seventieth anniversary would generate. Everything had been carefully curated. Bespoke, acid-free, grey boxes had been made for shoes and hats to ensure that they could be displayed without being touched and even a specially adapted hanger/suit carrier had been designed to avoid putting undue stress on delicate straps.

The centre was an absolute dream. We were shown treasures from the collection of over 250 outfits designed by Dior, and although we had seen an iconic Bar Suit in the exhibition – the black and white outfit ('Jupe plisée noire, fibranne/laine. Veste shantung grège soie.')

Left

Dior Heritage: the heritage centre is exceptional. The archive had not been of high priority and in some areas had glaring omissions. Prior to Dior's seventieth anniversary year in 2017, the archive received the attention it deserved. It had been moved from the original ateliers at 30 Avenue Montaigne into a purpose-built centre, ready to welcome the international interest that the anniversary would generate.

Right

Despite their late arrival at Blenheim, the mannequins were in time to enjoy a buffet supper at the reception held for them in the Great Hall. They tucked into chicken, hams, game and fruit before being whisked off to their host families.

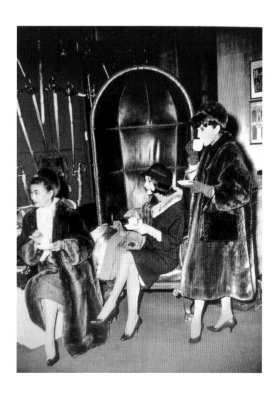

upon which each new creative director is obliged to base their first design – it was a real treat to see the one on display in the heritage centre at such close quarters. Soïzic explained that every haute couture outfit is still available today: it is simply a question of commission. I live in hope...

My daughters and I had tickets for a very late train back to the UK and originally thought we might do a spot of Christmas shopping after visiting the exhibition, but by now we had had had no lunch, no coffee and the effects of the early morning croissant provided by my daughter at St Pancras had long since worn off. All thoughts of shopping forgotten, we hunted down an Italian restaurant (I have a slight bias) and had a quick supper and a glass of

wine before heading back to the Gare du Nord and boarding our train. It had been the most amazing day.

A footnote: I was keen to give Soïzic a small token of my appreciation and, as well as a small selection of goodies from the Blenheim Gift Shop, I had managed to source a book written by Dior and first published in 1954, *The Little Dictionary of Fashion*. I was very excited to present her with it and did so just before we were given our tour. She received it with good grace and seemed pleased to do so. And then she opened one of the boxes she had put out to show us, which contained at least another half dozen of these books in several different languages!

Not such an inspired gift after all!

CHAPTER 13

Here comes the (Blenheim) bride

'A [bride] should be two things:
classy and fabulous'

—*Coco Chanel*

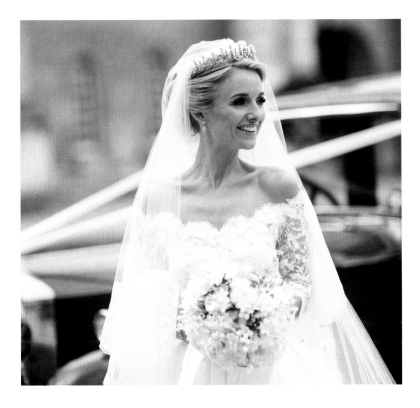

There have been many Blenheim brides, some beautiful, some joyous, some full of apprehension, sorrow or resignation. A windy September day in 2018 saw the most recent, and possibly the most romantic, Marlborough marriage. It was between George Blandford* the eldest son of the 12th Duke of Marlborough, and his childhood sweetheart, Camilla Thorp.

To date, there have been twelve Dukes of Marlborough including the present incumbent;

*The title Lord Blandford has for some time been that given to the eldest son of the Dukes of Marlborough. Upon succeeding to the dukedom, the holder of the title becomes the Duke of Marlborough and the title of Lord Blandford continues to be passed down. Although the family name is Spencer-Churchill, 'Marlborough' or 'Blandford' is used as a last name by the Duke and Duchess of Marlborough and by Lord and Lady Blandford respectively.

actually, that is not quite true as the second 'duke' – Henrietta Churchill – was female and a duchess in her own right. This unique and unparalleled situation came about because, at the time of his death, John Churchill, the 1st Duke of Marlborough, had no male heir. It was a mark of the great esteem and affection in which he and his wife were held by Queen Anne (until it all went horribly wrong) that an Act of Parliament had been passed allowing the Marlborough title to pass to and through the female line.

Putting Henrietta Churchill and her husband, Francis Godolphin, to one side for the moment, it has to be said that, through reasons of death or divorce, there have been far more duchesses, dowager duchesses or duchesses-in-waiting in Blenheim Palace's 300-year history than there have been dukes.

The 1st Duke and Duchess, Sarah and John
Churchill, are said to have been married
secretly sometime in 1678, possibly so that
Sarah could continue at court as a Maid
of Honour, one of the requirements of this
much-coveted position being that the holders
should be 'maids' in the true sense of the word.
We have no record of what the bride wore on
that occasion, but subsequent duchesses and
other family members are known to have
been dressed in the best that money and good
taste could buy. Gladys Deacon, who married
the newly divorced 9th Duke in 1921, took
things a step further when she spearheaded
an advertising campaign by Pond's in which
an image of her dressed in her exquisite ivory
lace wedding gown was used to promote their
famous face creams.

For Consuelo Vanderbilt's first marriage,
her mother Alva had had the foresight to order
a wedding gown from the House of Worth
in Paris, long before the 9th Duke actually
made his proposal. For her second marriage,
to Jacques Balsan, French aviator and love of
her life, Consuelo was more modestly dressed
in a silver silk gown, plain black hat and a
single string of 'glorious' pearls at her throat.
Among the guests on this happy occasion (no
tears from the bride this time) was Consuelo's
daughter-in-law, later the 10th Duchess. She
favoured British designer Hardy Amies, whom
she commissioned to dress her youngest
daughter, Lady Rosemary, when she married
in 1953. Lady Rosemary had postponed her
marriage to act as a Maid of Honour to HM
Queen Elizabeth II at her coronation: an echo
of her ancestor Sarah's wish not to let her
nuptials interfere with duties at court perhaps?

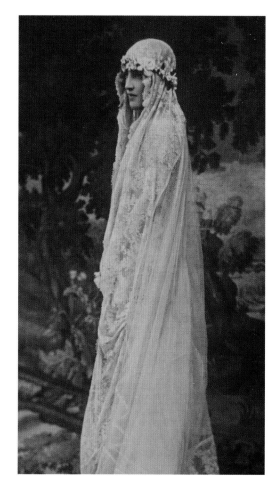

Above
Gladys Deacon, who
married the newly
divorced 9th Duke in
1921, spearheaded an
advertising campaign by
Pond's in which an image of
her dressed in her exquisite
ivory lace wedding gown
was used to promote its
famous face creams.

Once the Blandford and Thorp engagement was announced early in December 2017, preparations for the perfect Blenheim wedding celebration began. The venue was secured – not quite as simple as you might think given the number of celebrations held at the Palace, many of them booked years in advance – and everything else fell into place beautifully.

George and Camilla's marriage, the latest thread in the tapestry of Blenheim's wedding history, was a marvellous blend of historic and modern from the very beginning. Their romance began on the Isle of Wight, as did that of an earlier Marlborough notable, Lord Randolph (father of the famous – but oh so unstylish – Winston), but fortunately the prospect of this most recent union was greeted with delight by all concerned, unlike that of

Randolph Churchill and Jennie Jerome.

Continuing the historic theme, Camilla wore for her wedding an heirloom that has been in the Marlborough family since 1895: the Boucheron tiara, which was literally sewn into her hair, had originally been a wedding gift to Consuelo Vanderbilt from her father. Consuelo refers to the diamond tiara capped with pearls in her memoir, but speaks of it with little affection, describing only the 'violent headache' it invariably produced when she wore it. Perhaps that is why she eventually presented it to Alexandra Mary Cadogan, later the 10th Duchess, on the occasion of her wedding to Consuelo's eldest son 'Bert'. Fortunately, Camilla's memories of wearing it are significantly happier and she found it both light and comfortable.

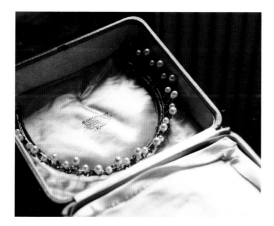

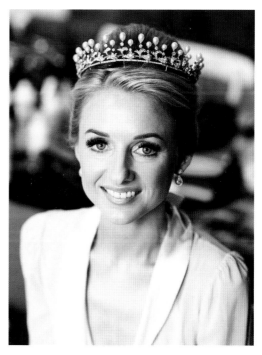

Above
The Boucheron tiara, which has been in the Marlborough family since 1895. It was originally a wedding gift to Consuelo Vanderbilt from her father.

Right
The tiara was literally sewn into Lady Blandford's hair. Fortunately, her memories of wearing it are significantly happier than Consuelo's ever were.

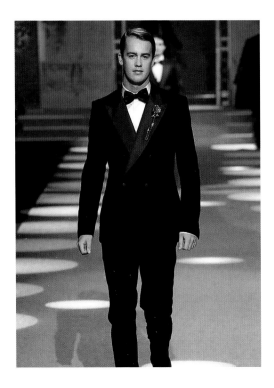

Italian designers, this being the first wedding dress created for a bride in the UK.

Like all brides, Camilla considered various options before selecting a designer for her wedding gown. For her, the ability of Domenico Dolce and Stefano Gabbana to clothe a woman in exquisite style and femininity won the day. Camilla was closely involved in the design of both her wedding gown and a second dress for the evening. In response to her own likes and instinct for what suited her, alongside the suggestions of the designers, she decided upon the character and features of the fabric to be used in the creation of both dresses.

A second meeting in Milan saw Camilla being presented with bespoke samples of fabrics for the flowing wedding dress and also for the corseted evening dress that she would change into after the formalities of the day. The wearing of a corset was perhaps an echo of the style of many earlier Lady Blandfords, but again a far more comfortable experience, without the damaging effects of prolonged use suffered by the earlier ladies.

On this occasion the exact measurements of every centimetre of Camilla's figure were taken. These were then used to create a bespoke monogrammed mannequin upon which the dress could be constructed and which would reflect her shape so precisely that, when she had her final fitting just two days before the wedding, the dress needed only 'a couple of tweaks' for it to fit like a glove.

And so, nine months after becoming engaged, on Saturday 8 September, Camilla arrived at St Mary Magdalene's Church, Woodstock, dressed in her exquisite wedding gown. The off-the-shoulder bodice was of lace, embellished with tiny pale pink and white

But what about the dress! Every bride wants to look her best on her wedding day and knows that she will be the centre of attention. George Blandford is a very stylish young man by anyone's standards and, like his great-uncle Charles before him, is known in the world of fashion. Lord Charles Spencer-Churchill lent his name to a line of menswear in the US – the Lord Charles Churchill Line – while Lord George 'walked' for Dolce & Gabbana in their Millennial Show in Milan in 2018. Perhaps knowing this, and with the additional pressure created by social media (most of her predecessors had only the press to worry about at worst), Camilla realised that 'classy and fabulous' was a must. It has to be said that, with her D&G gown, she got it absolutely right, and at the same time made fashion history for the

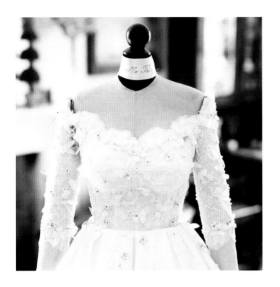

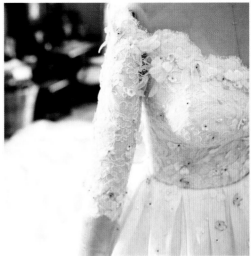

Left
Lord Blandford 'walked' for Dolce & Gabbana in their Millennial Show in Milan in 2018.

Above
Exact measurements of Lady Blandford's figure were taken. From these Dolce & Gabbana created a bespoke monogrammed mannequin upon which the dress could be fitted.

Above right
The off-the-shoulder bodice was of lace, embellished with tiny pale pink and white appliquéd flowers and seed pearls, which then continued onto the skirt.

Below
Newly-weds George and Camilla Blandford pictured in Blenheim's Great Court.

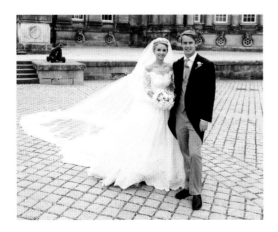

appliquéd flowers and seed pearls, which then continued onto the skirt. The skirt itself was made up of layers of tulle for volume and topped with a layer of organza. The delicate lace featured again both on the hem of the skirt and around the edge of the silk tulle veil secured by the tiara. The complete picture was of a happy, smiling bride. No sorrow, no apprehension, no resignation, just beauty and pure, radiant joy.

The 10th Duchess once remarked that, 'All those who come to be connected with Blenheim feel a pride that they never really lose'. It is rather splendid to think that this observation is still true today and seems to apply as much to one of Duchess Mary's successors – Camilla Blandford – as it did in 1920, when she herself married into this most remarkable family.

Index

Picture credits

All photographs by Richard Cragg, Blenheim Palace or author's own unless otherwise stated

Cover photograph: Willy Rizzo@Archives Paris Match; p.8 Victoria & Albert Museum; p.16 Churchill wedding – unknown; p.16 © Hugo Vickers; p.19 Macaroni By Philip Dawe - Amelia F[aye] Rauser (Autumn 2004). "Hair, Authenticity, and the Self-Made Macaroni". Eighteenth-Century Studies 38 (1): 101–117 at 106., Public Domain, https://commons.wikimedia.org/w/index.php?curid=12087243; p.22 Topham Beauclerk – unknown; p.25 © Denise Watson; p.38 Sciencephoto.com; p.39 Coiffure à l'échelle. Caricature du XVIII siècle – Getty images; p.44 Gunning cartoon – By James Gillray https://commons.wikimedia.org/w/index.php?curid=6370759; p.49 Georgiana Duchess of Devonshire - By Thomas Gainsborough - Unknown, Public Domain, https://commons.wikimedia.org/w/index.php?curid=670042; p.55 Running Footman – Alamy; p 60 Christian Davies – unknown; p.65 Winding up the Ladies – Alamy; p.75 Arsenic Waltz - https://commons.wikimedia.org/w/index.php?curid=36648437; p.76 Miss Prattle consulting Dr Double Fee - Alamy; p.77 Wasp waist - Unknown - Victoria and Albert Museum, Public Domain https://commons.wikimedia.org/w/index.php?curid=31236607; p.78 Cruikshank Crinoline parody - By George Cruikshank - The Comic Almanack for 1850 (Scanned by H. Churchyard), Public Domain, https://commons.wikimedia.org/w/index.php?curid=550206; p.79 Arsenic Gown – unknown; p.81 Mad Hatter - By John Tenniel - vector version of Image:MadlHatterByTenniel.jpg), public domain, https://commons.wikimedia.org/w/index.php?curid=5074817; P84 Blenheim Palace by Pete Seaward; p.103 The Princess of Wales at the Braemar Games 1981 – Getty images; p.112 © Christina Stambolian; p.113 © Christina Stambolian; Christian Dior – Quite a Revolution; p.117 The 10th Duchess as a 21 year old – © Lady Rosemary Muir; p.119 sketch for the 'Margaret' dress. Dior Héritage collection, Paris; p120 Princess Margaret photographed by Cecil Beaton. The Victoria and Albert Museum; p.124 Victoria & Albert Museum; p.132 Adrien Dirand, Dior Héritage collection, Paris; p.135 Matt Porteous; p.136 © Hugo Vickers; p.137 Tiara - Matt Porteous; p.137 Tiara on - Matt Porteous; p.138 not known; p.139 all by Matt Porteous;

Acknowledgements

None of this would have been possible without the generous help and encouragement of:

The Duke and Duchess of Marlborough
Lord and Lady Blandford
Lady Rosemary Muir
Richard Cragg
Christina Stambolian
Svetlana Lloyd
Dior Héritage

Dominic Hare and Heather Carter for trusting me with the *A Passion for Fashion* exhibition and for having faith in this project.

My splendid colleagues at Blenheim Palace for whom nothing was too much trouble.

The team at Unicorn Publishing Group

Constant 'radiator' Alison Derham never a drain!

Bernadette Allison.

Gerry, my long suffering, endlessly patient and loving husband.

...and, last but never least,

Amy, Rachel and Dilly, our three daughters and little Mia Antonia Jane Ford – the very latest addition to the Family of Five (Plus!).

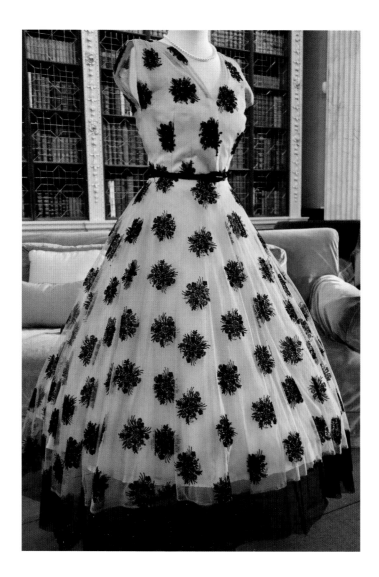

Above
A beautiful black and white
1950s dress - in the style of
Christian Dior

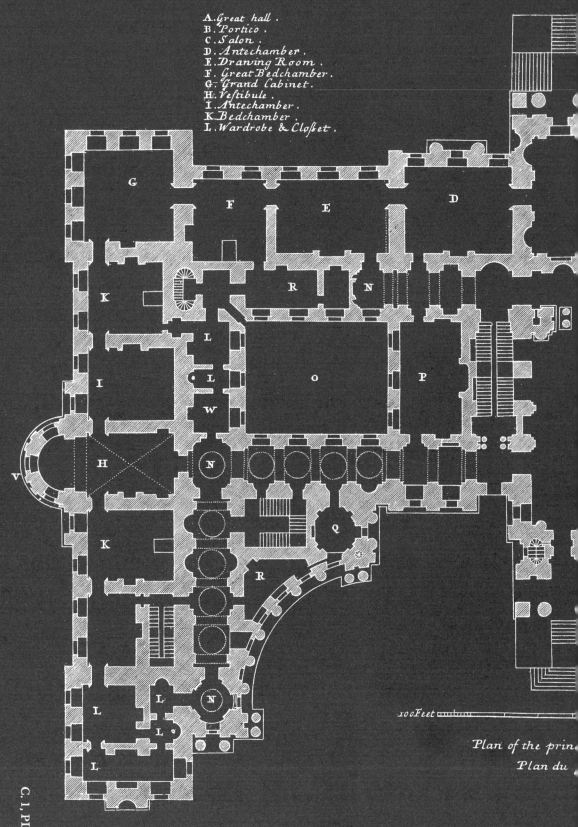

A. *Great hall* .
B. *Portico* .
C. *Salon* .
D. *Antechamber* .
E. *Drawing Room* .
F. *Great Bedchamber* .
G. *Grand Cabinet* .
H. *Vestibule* .
I. *Antechamber* .
K. *Bedchamber* .
L. *Wardrobe & Closet* .

100 Feet

Plan of the prin

Plan du